The Essential Dash Diet Cookbook

-The Ultimate Cookbook to Decrease Hypertension by Reducing Sodium, Saturated Fat and Excess Sugars with Recipes that Practically Cook Themselves -

[Sebastian Osborne]

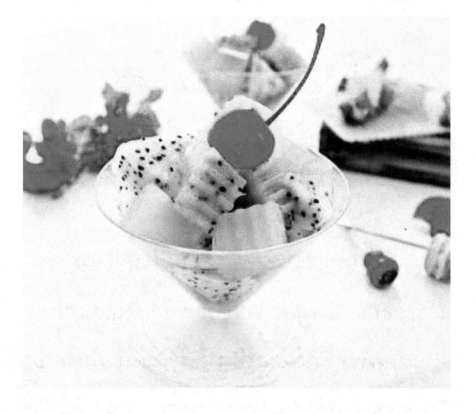

Table Of Content

5

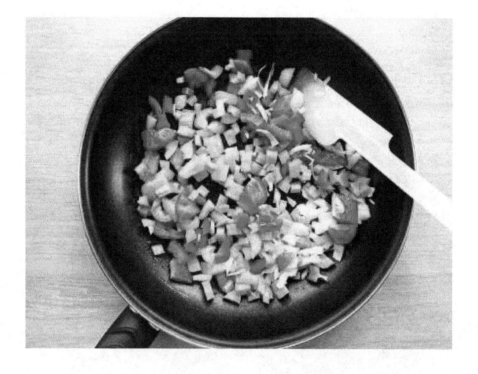

Additionally, the information in the following pages is intended only for informational purposes and should thus be thought of as universal. As befitting its nature, it is presented without assurance regarding its prolonged validity or interim quality. Trademarks that are mentioned are done without written consent and can in no way be considered an endorsement from the trademark holder.

CHAPTER 1: BREAKFAST

Vegan Muesli

Prep:

10 mins

Additional:

8 hrs

Total:

8 hrs 10 mins

Servings:

6

Yield:

6 servings

Ingredients

2 cups rolled oats

3 tablespoons chia seeds

2 Granny Smith apples, peeled and grated

½ lemon, juiced

1 ½ (14 ounce) cans coconut milk

1 cup blueberries

2 tablespoons maple syrup

2 cups sliced strawberries

Directions

1

Mix oats, coconut milk, and chia seeds together in a bowl.

2

Toss apples and lemon juice together in a bowl until coated; fold into oat mixture. Stir strawberries, blueberries, and maple syrup into oat mixture. Refrigerate for 8 hours to overnight.

Nutrition

Per Serving: 392 calories; protein 7.1g; carbohydrates 42.2g; fat 24.6g; sodium 17.5mg.

Moming Quinoa

Prep:

5 mins

Cook:

35 mins

Total:

40 mins

Servings:

2

Yield:

2 servings

Ingredients

2 cups chicken broth

2 tablespoons olive oil

2 cloves garlic, minced

1 cup quinoa

1 small onion, diced

1 tablespoon ancho chile powder

salt and pepper to taste

1 tablespoon curry powder

Directions

1

Heat oil in a large skillet over medium heat. Add onion and garlic and cook and stir for 2 minutes; add quinoa and cook and stir until lightly toasted, about 5-6 minutes.

2

Pour broth into the pan and bring to a boil. Reduce heat and add curry and chile powders; cover and simmer until tender, about 25 minutes. Season to taste with salt and pepper.

Nutrition

Per Serving: 473 calories; protein 13.5g; carbohydrates 62.8g; fat 19.8g; sodium 48.2mg

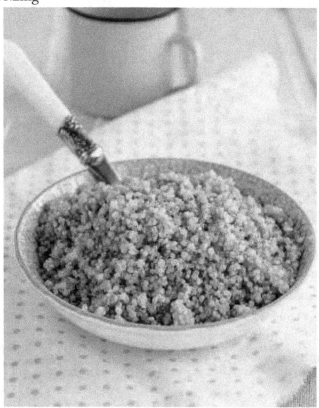

Baked Oatmeal

Prep:

10 mins

Cook:

40 mins

Total:

50 mins

Servings:

8

Yield:

8 servings

Ingredients

3 cups rolled oats

¾ cup brown sugar

2 teaspoons ground cinnamon (such as McCormick® Roasted Saigon Cinnamon)

1 teaspoon salt

1 cup milk

½ cup melted butter

2 teaspoons baking powder

2 eggs

2 teaspoons vanilla extract

¼ cup dried cranberries

¼ cup maple syrup

Directions

1

Preheat oven to 350 degrees F. Grease an 8x8-inch baking dish.

2

Mix oats, brown sugar, cinnamon, baking powder, and salt together in a bowl. Beat in milk, butter, maple syrup, eggs, and vanilla extract; fold in cranberries. Spread mixture into the prepared baking dish.

3

Bake in the preheated oven until bubbling, about 40 minutes.

Nutrition

Per Serving: 344 calories; protein 6.7g; carbohydrates 46g; fat 15.4g; cholesterol 79.4mg; sodium 531mg.

Banana Nut Pancakes

Prep:

15 mins

Cook:

4 mins

Total:

19 mins

Servings:

3

Yield:

6 to 8 pancakes

Ingredients

1 cup all-purpose flour

¼ cup finely chopped walnuts

1 tablespoon baking powder

½ teaspoon ground nutmeg

½ teaspoon ground cinnamon

3 tablespoons white sugar

½ teaspoon baking soda

½ teaspoon salt

2 small overripe bananas, mashed

1 ½ tablespoons butter, melted

1 cup almond milk

½ teaspoon vanilla extract

1 egg

Directions

1

Mix flour, walnuts, sugar, baking powder, nutmeg, cinnamon, baking soda, and salt in a large bowl; make a well in the center.

2

Whisk almond milk, bananas, melted butter, and vanilla extract together in a separate bowl until smooth. Whisk in egg. Pour mixture into the well in the flour mixture; stir until just combined.

3

Heat a lightly oiled skillet over medium-high heat. Drop 1/4 cup batter into the skillet; tilt gently to spread batter evenly. Cook until bubbles form and the edges are firm, 3 to 4 minutes. Flip and cook until browned on the other side, 1 to 3 minutes more. Repeat with remaining batter.

Nutrition

Per Serving: 427 calories; protein 9.1g; carbohydrates 65.5g; fat 15.5g; cholesterol 77.3mg; sodium 1052.4mg.

Fruit Pizza

Prep:

15 mins

Cook:

5 mins

Additional:

30 mins

Total:

50 mins

Servings:

8

Yield:

8 servings

Ingredients

Crust:

1 cup crushed cornflakes

2 tablespoons light corn syrup

2 tablespoons white sugar

2 tablespoons butter, softened

1 tablespoon honey

Frosting:

2 (8 ounce) packages cream cheese, softened

1 (7 ounce) jar marshmallow fluff

Toppings:

½ cup sliced strawberries

2 kiwi, peeled and sliced

2 apricots, sliced

Directions

1

Preheat oven to 350 degrees F.

2

Mix cornflakes, butter, corn syrup, and sugar in a bowl until evenly combined; press onto a baking sheet.

3

Bake in the preheated oven until crust is golden brown, about 5 minutes. Drizzle crust with honey and cool in refrigerator, about 15-17 minutes.

4

Stir cream cheese and marshmallow fluff together in a bowl until smooth and creamy; spread over cooled crust, keeping a 1/2-inch border of crust. Chill crust in refrigerator until completely cooled, about 15 minutes.

5

Arrange strawberries, apricots, and kiwi over the cream cheese layer.

Nutrition

Per Serving: 366 calories; protein 5.1g; carbohydrates 37.6g; fat 22.7g; cholesterol 69.2mg; sodium 235.1mg.

J Yogurt

Prep:

10 mins

Additional:

2 hrs

Total:

2 hrs 10 mins

Servings:

6

Yield:

6 servings

Ingredients

1 cup plain Greek yogurt

2 tablespoons natural peanut butter

¼ cup mashed strawberries

1 tablespoon maple syrup

4 fresh strawberries, sliced

2 teaspoons natural peanut butter

¼ teaspoon vanilla extract

1 teaspoon coconut oil

Directions

1

Mix yogurt, mashed strawberries, 2 tablespoons peanut butter, maple syrup, and vanilla extract together in a bowl.

2

Line a baking sheet with parchment paper and spread yogurt mixture in a thin layer onto the parchment paper. Top mixture with sliced strawberries.

3

Stir 2 teaspoons peanut butter and coconut oil together in a microwave-safe bowl; heat in microwave until melted, about 30 seconds. Stir well and drizzle over yogurt mixture.

4

Freeze yogurt mixture until solid, at least 2 hours. Break into pieces.

Nutrition

Per Serving: 108 calories; protein 3.8g; carbohydrates 6.8g; fat 7.7g; cholesterol 7.5mg; sodium 39.9mg.

Sweet Millet Congee

Prep:

20 mins

Cook:

3 hrs 15 mins

Total:

3 hrs 35 mins

Servings:

6

Yield:

6 servings

Ingredients

5 cups chicken stock

5 cups water

1 cup white rice

¼ cup apple cider vinegar

½ teaspoon vinegar

1 tablespoon grated fresh ginger

1 teaspoon salt

2 tablespoons fish sauce

2 (6 ounce) fillets lean white fish, sliced

¼ cup sliced Chinese roast pork

2 tablespoons chopped scallions

¼ teaspoon sesame oil

2 tablespoons crushed peanuts

¼ cup pickled Chinese vegetables

½ teaspoon soy sauce

Directions

1

Combine chicken stock, water, rice, 1/4 cup apple cider vinegar, fish sauce, ginger, salt, and sesame oil in a large stockpot; bring to a boil. Reduce heat and simmer until congee has thickened to the consistency of a light porridge, about 3 hours.

2

Stir fish into congee and simmer until cooked through, about 10-12 minutes.

3

Serve congee in bowls topped with pickled vegetables, roast pork, scallions, and peanuts. Drizzle 1/2 teaspoon vinegar and soy sauce over toppings.

Nutrition

Per Serving: 205 calories; protein 15.1g; carbohydrates 28.3g; fat 2.9g; cholesterol 25.4mg; sodium 1430.7mg.

Sunrise Smoothies

Prep:

15 mins

Total:

15 mins

Servings:

2

Yield:

2 servings

Ingredients

½ cup orange juice

1 teaspoon white sugar

1 banana, frozen and chunked

½ cup honeydew melon, cubed

1 (8 ounce) container orange yogurt

1 peach, peeled and sliced

½ cup ice

Directions

1

Combine the orange juice, banana, peach, honeydew melon, yogurt, sugar, and ice in a blender. Blend until smooth, or chunky, as desired. Pour into two glasses and serve.

Nutrition

Per Serving: 239 calories; protein 5.8g; carbohydrates 52g; fat 1.3g; cholesterol 9mg; sodium 67.4mg.

Breakfast Bread Pudding

Prep:

25 mins

Cook:

45 mins

Additional:

8 hrs 5 mins

Total:

9 hrs 15 mins

Servings:

12

Yield:

1 9x13-inch baking dish

Ingredients

6 eggs

1 cup milk

1 teaspoon ground cinnamon

½ cup heavy cream

1 tablespoon vanilla extract

1 (16 ounce) loaf cinnamon bread with raisins, cut into 1-inch cubes

2 Granny Smith apples - peeled, cored, and sliced

1 teaspoon ground nutmeg

1 cup brown sugar

¼ cup melted butter

1 Granny Smith apple - peeled, cored, and diced

Directions

1

Beat the eggs in a mixing bowl. Whisk in the milk, cream, vanilla extract, and nutmeg until evenly blended. Fold in the bread cubes and set aside until the bread soaks up the egg mixture, about 5 minutes. Place the sliced apples into a mixing bowl and sprinkle with brown sugar, cinnamon, and melted butter; toss to evenly coat. Grease a 9x13-inch baking dish and arrange the apple slices evenly into the bottom of the prepared baking dish; spoon the bread mixture over top. Cover the dish with aluminum foil and refrigerate overnight.

2

Preheat an oven to 375 degrees F.

3

Sprinkle the diced apple over the bread pudding and cover again with the aluminum foil. Bake in the preheated oven until the bread is no longer soggy, about 40 minutes. Remove the foil and set the oven to Broil; broil until golden brown on top, about 5-6 minutes. Remove and let stand 5 to 10 minutes before serving.

Nutrition

Per Serving: 312 calories; protein 8.3g; carbohydrates 43g; fat 12.5g; cholesterol 118.4mg; sodium 221.7mg.

Green Smoothie

Prep:
5 mins
Total:
5 mins
Servings:
2
Yield:
2 smoothies

Ingredients

2 cups baby spinach
½ teaspoon chopped jalapeno pepper
1 cup frozen mango chunks
1 cup water
2 bananas, broken into chunks

Directions
1
Layer banana, spinach, mango, and jalapeno pepper in a blender; add water and blend until smooth, adding more water for a thinner smoothie.

Nutrition
Per Serving: 166 calories; protein 2.6g; carbohydrates 42.1g; fat 0.7g; sodium 30.1mg.

Jack-o-Lantern Pancakes

Prep:

10 mins

Cook:

10 mins

Total:

20 mins

Servings:

6

Yield:

6 servings

Ingredients

1 cup all-purpose flour

¼ cup brown sugar

2 teaspoons baking powder

¼ teaspoon ground cinnamon

¼ teaspoon ground cloves

1 cup quick cooking oats

½ teaspoon salt

¾ cup canned pumpkin

2 tablespoons vegetable oil

¾ cup semisweet chocolate chips

1 cup milk

1 egg, beaten

Directions

1

Stir together flour, oats, brown sugar, baking powder, cinnamon, cloves, and salt in a large bowl. In a separate large bowl, lightly beat together the milk, egg, pumpkin, and oil. Stir flour mixture into the pumpkin mixture, blending just until moistened.

2

Heat a lightly greased griddle over medium high heat.

3

Pour batter, 1/3 cup at a time, onto the prepared griddle. Make a jack-o-lantern face in each pancake with the chocolate chips. Cook until bubbles appear on the surface, then flip and cook until golden brown on the other side, about 5 minutes per side.

Nutrition

Per Serving: 347 calories; protein 7.6g; carbohydrates 52.3g; fat 13.7g; cholesterol 34.3mg; sodium 464.8mg.

Flax Banana Muffins

Prep:

10 mins

Cook:

20 mins

Total:

30 mins

Servings:

20

Yield:

20 muffins

Ingredients

6 large ripe bananas

1 cup brown sugar

½ cup white sugar

2 eggs

1 ½ cups all-purpose flour

¾ cup salted butter, melted

1 ¼ cups whole wheat flour

2 teaspoons baking soda

2 teaspoons baking powder

½ cup ground flax seeds

Directions

1

Preheat oven to 350 degrees F. Line 2 muffin tins with paper liners.

2

Mash bananas in a bowl. Add brown sugar, butter, white sugar, and eggs; mix well. Add all-purpose flour, whole wheat flour, flax seeds, baking soda, and baking powder. Scoop batter into the prepared tins.

3

Bake in the preheated oven until tops spring back when lightly pressed, about 20-22 minutes.

Nutrition

Per Serving: 240 calories; protein 3.7g; carbohydrates 38.7g; fat 8.9g; cholesterol 36.9mg; sodium 235.5mg.

Sweet Potato Cakes

Prep:

10 mins

Cook:

25 mins

Additional:

30 mins

Total:

1 hr 5 mins

Servings:

12

Yield:

12 servings

Ingredients

2 ¾ cups all-purpose flour

1 cup white sugar

¼ cup sweet potato puree

2 teaspoons ground cinnamon

½ teaspoon salt

¼ teaspoon ground cloves

1 ¾ cups cooled coffee

1 ½ teaspoons baking powder

¾ cup olive oil

Icing:

1 cup confectioners' sugar

1 teaspoon vanilla extract

¼ teaspoon ground cinnamon

1 tablespoon orange juice

Directions

1

Preheat the oven to 350 degrees F. Grease a 9x13-inch baking pan.

2

Combine flour, sugar, cinnamon, baking powder, salt, and cloves in a bowl and mix well. Add cooled coffee, oil, and sweet potato puree; mix well. Pour batter evenly into the prepared baking pan.

3

Bake in the preheated oven until a toothpick inserted in the center comes out clean, 25 to 30 minutes. Remove and allow to cool on a wire rack, about 30 minutes.

4

Stir together 1 cup confectioners' sugar, 1 tablespoon orange juice, vanilla extract, and cinnamon in a bowl. Add more sugar or orange juice, if needed, to achieve your desired consistency. Drizzle icing over the top of the cooled cake.

Nutrition

Per Serving: 336 calories; protein 3.1g; carbohydrates 50.4g; fat 13.8g; sodium 163.7mg.

Orange-Blueberry Muffin

Prep:

25 mins

Cook:

15 mins

Additional:

20 mins

Total:

1 hr

Servings:

12

Yield:

12 muffins

Ingredients

½ cup oat bran

1 cup wheat bran

½ cup sour cream

1 cup all-purpose flour

1 teaspoon baking powder

1 teaspoon baking soda

½ cup milk

⅔ cup brown sugar

½ teaspoon salt

⅓ cup vegetable oil

1 orange, juiced and zested

1 cup fresh blueberries

1 egg

1 teaspoon vanilla extract

Directions

1

Preheat an oven to 375 degrees F. Grease 12 muffin cups, or line with paper muffin liners.

2

Combine the oat bran and wheat bran in a large bowl. Stir in sour cream and milk. Allow mixture to stand for 10 minutes. Combine flour, baking powder, baking soda, brown sugar, and salt in a separate bowl. Gently stir blueberries into the flour mixture, carefully coating all the blueberries with flour. Stir vegetable oil, orange juice and zest, egg, and vanilla extract into the bran mixture. Combine flour mixture with the wet ingredients until just blended. Drop batter into lined muffin cups.

3

Bake in the preheated oven until a toothpick inserted into the center comes out clean, 15 to 20 minutes. Cool in the pans for 10 minutes before removing to cool completely on a wire rack.

Nutrition

Per Serving: 182 calories; protein 3.8g; carbohydrates 24.4g; fat 9.3g; cholesterol 20.5mg; sodium 260.4mg.

Warmed Stuffed Peaches

Prep:

20 mins

Cook:

10 mins

Additional:

8 hrs

Total:

8 hrs 30 mins

Servings:

4

Yield:

4 servings

Ingredients

Dressing:

1 medium red bell pepper, chopped

½ teaspoon garlic paste

¼ cup chopped yellow onion

2 tablespoons vegetable oil

2 tablespoons honey

¼ cup apple cider vinegar

½ teaspoon freshly grated ginger

Salad:

1 tablespoon vegetable oil

½ pound kale leaves, veins removed

⅓ cup goat cheese

2 peaches, each cut into 8 wedges

salt and pepper to taste

Directions

1

Combine red bell pepper, vinegar, onion, oil, honey, ginger, and garlic paste in a jar with a lid. Cover jar, shake, and refrigerate dressing 8 hours to overnight.

2

Preheat an outdoor grill for medium-high heat and lightly oil the grate.

3

Place peaches and kale on the preheated grill. Toss kale continuously until softened and lightly charred on the edges, about 5 minutes. Cook and turn peaches until grill marks appear, about 3 minutes per side.

4

Place cooked kale in a serving bowl and toss with dressing. Top with cooked peaches and goat cheese. Season with salt and pepper. Serve warm.

Nutrition

Per Serving: 223 calories; protein 4.8g; carbohydrates 20.5g; fat 14.2g; cholesterol 9.2mg; sodium 149.3mg.

Tropical Fruit Parfaits

Prep:

5 mins

Total:

5 mins

Servings:

4

Yield:

4 servings

Ingredients

2 cups vanilla yogurt
2 cups mixed fresh berries (raspberries, blueberries, strawberries), hulled and sliced
2 cups granola

Directions

1

Set out yogurt, granola, and berries in bowls with serving spoons. Let each person layer their own parfaits in cups or glasses.

Nutrition

Per Serving: 429 calories; protein 15.7g; carbohydrates 55.8g; fat 16.5g; cholesterol 6.1mg; sodium 96.9mg.

Multigrain Pancakes

Prep:

10 mins

Cook:

15 mins

Total:

25 mins

Servings:

4

Yield:

4 servings

Ingredients

¼ cup whole wheat flour

¼ cup all-purpose flour

½ teaspoon baking soda

¼ cup rolled oats

¼ cup cornmeal

½ teaspoon salt

1 teaspoon baking powder

½ teaspoon ground cinnamon

2 egg whites

2 tablespoons plain nonfat yogurt

2 tablespoons skim milk

2 teaspoons granular no-calorie sucralose sweetener (e.g., Splenda ®)

2 tablespoons water

Directions

1

In a medium bowl, stir together the whole wheat flour, all-purpose flour, oats, cornmeal, sweetener, salt, baking powder, baking soda and cinnamon. In a separate bowl, whisk together the eggs, yogurt, milk and water. Pour the wet ingredients into the dry, and mix just until moistened.

2

Heat a skillet over medium heat, and coat with cooking spray. Pour about 1/3 cup of batter per pancake onto the skillet. Cook until bubbles begin to form in the center, then flip and cook until browned on the other side.

Nutrition

Per Serving: 120 calories; protein 5.5g; carbohydrates 23.2g; fat 0.7g; cholesterol 0.3mg; sodium 574.8mg.

Quinoa Pancakes

Prep:

10 mins

Cook:

5 mins

Total:

15 mins

Servings:

10

Yield:

10 servings

Ingredients

1 ½ cups quinoa flour

2 tablespoons honey

1 ½ teaspoons baking powder

½ teaspoon salt

3 eggs, beaten

2 tablespoons butter, melted

1 ¼ cups flaxseed milk

Directions

1

Grease a griddle or large skillet and preheat over medium heat.

2

Stir quinoa flour, baking powder, and salt together in a bowl. Stir flaxseed milk, eggs, melted butter, and honey into the flour mixture until you have a thin batter.

3

Pour 1/4 cup batter onto your hot cooking surface per pancake and cook until bubbles form on top, 2 to 3 minutes. Flip the pancake and cook until browned on the bottom, about 2 minutes more.

Nutrition

Per Serving: 138 calories; protein 4.9g; carbohydrates 17.3g; fat 5.6g; cholesterol 61.9mg; sodium 241.1mg.

Spiced Oatmeal

Prep:

5 mins

Cook:

2 mins

Total:

7 mins

Servings:

1

Yield:

1 serving

Ingredients

¾ cup old-fashioned rolled oats

½ cup frozen blueberries

1 cup water

¼ cup orange juice

½ teaspoon ground cinnamon

¼ cup dried cranberries

Directions

1

Place the rolled oats, cinnamon, cranberries, and blueberries in a microwave safe bowl. Add the turmeric and ginger, if desired. Pour in the water, and stir to mix ingredients. Cook on High until water is absorbed, about 2 minutes. Stir in orange juice to desired consistency.

Nutrition

Per Serving: 398 calories; protein 9.1g; carbohydrates 84.8g; fat 4.5g; sodium 12.7mg.

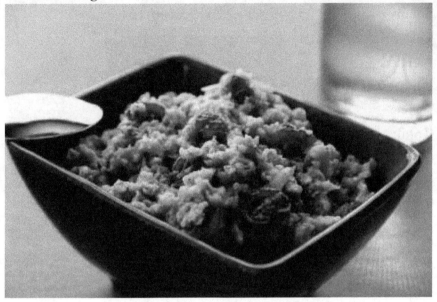

Maple Oatmeal

Prep:

5 mins

Cook:

6 mins

Additional:

2 mins

Total:

13 mins

Servings:

1

Yield:

1 serving

Ingredients

1 ½ cups water

1 tablespoon maple syrup

1 tablespoon packed dark brown sugar

¾ cup quick-cooking oats

Directions

1

Bring water to a boil. Add oats and cook, stirring, for 1 minute. Remove from heat and stir in brown sugar and maple syrup. Let sit until desired thickness is reached, 2 to 4 minutes.

Nutrition

Per Serving: 334 calories; protein 8g; carbohydrates 67.9g; fat 4g; sodium 19.9mg.

The Dipper

Prep:

20 mins

Cook:

20 mins

Total:

40 mins

Servings:

8

Yield:

4 sandwiches

Ingredients

1 onion, sliced

1 tablespoon garlic basil spread

1 tablespoon Italian seasoning

1 cup sliced mushrooms

2 tablespoons Marsala wine

1 cup beef broth

2 pounds sliced roast beef

1 cup pickled sweet and hot pepper rings

4 ciabatta sandwich rolls, sliced horizontally

1 tablespoon olive oil

¼ cup prepared horseradish sauce, divided

12 slices Swiss cheese, divided

¼ cup garlic basil spread, divided

Directions

1

Preheat oven to 500 degrees F.

2

Heat olive oil in a large pot or Dutch oven over medium heat. Cook and stir onion, 1 tablespoon garlic basil spread, and Italian seasoning in the hot oil until onion has softened, 4 to 6 minutes. Stir in pepper rings and mushrooms; cook and stir until mushrooms have softened, about 5 minutes.

3

Pour in Marsala wine and bring to a boil, scraping up any browned bits from the bottom of the pan. Add beef broth and roast beef and stir until the beef is warmed through, approximately 4 minutes.

4

Spread each ciabatta roll with 1 tablespoon garlic basil spread and 1 tablespoon horseradish sauce. Top with 3 slices Swiss cheese.

5

Place sandwiches on a baking sheet and bake in the preheated oven until the cheese is melted and the bread is toasted, 3 to 5 minutes. Using a slotted spoon, pile the beef-onion mixture into each sandwich and pour 1 to 2 tablespoons pan juices over the filling. Transfer the remaining pan juices to small bowls for dipping.

Nutrition

Per Serving: 976 calories; protein 55.5g; carbohydrates 123.1g; fat 28.4g; cholesterol 93.7mg; sodium 2723mg.

Light Biscuits

Prep:

15 mins

Cook:

20 mins

Total:

35 mins

Servings:

16

Yield:

16 servings

Ingredients

4 cups all-purpose flour

8 ounces crumbled cooked bacon

1 ½ cups butter, cut into large chunks

1 ¾ cups buttermilk

¼ cup baking powder

Directions

1

Preheat oven to 350 degrees F. Lightly butter 2 muffin tins.

2

Mix flour and baking powder together in a large bowl; cut in butter until mixture resembles coarse crumbs. Stir buttermilk and bacon into flour mixture just until dough holds together.

3

Turn dough onto a floured surface and roll into an even thickness. Fold dough over itself a few times. Cut dough into circles using a cookie or biscuit cutter and arrange circles in the prepared muffin tins.

4

Bake in the preheated oven on the top rack until biscuits are lightly browned, about 23-25 minutes.

Nutrition

Per Serving: 355 calories; protein 9.6g; carbohydrates 26g; fat 23.7g; cholesterol 62.4mg; sodium 746.8mg.

Honey-Ginger Kale Salad

Prep:

30 mins

Total:

30 mins

Servings:

6

Yield:

6 servings

Ingredients

2 tablespoons cider vinegar

2 (10 ounce) bunches lacinato kale, stems removed, leaves thinly sliced

1 ½ teaspoons low-sodium soy sauce

1 ½ teaspoons grated fresh ginger

2 tablespoons olive oil

1 ½ tablespoons fresh orange juice

1 ½ teaspoons honey

Directions

1

Whisk together vinegar, juice, soy sauce, honey, and ginger in a small bowl. Add oil slowly, whisking constantly until incorporated.

2

Put kale in a large bowl. Drizzle with dressing, and mix well. Using your hands, massage kale until softened, wilted, and reduced in volume by about half.

Nutrition

Per Serving: 89 calories; protein 2.8g; carbohydrates 10g; fat 5.1g; sodium 110.9mg.

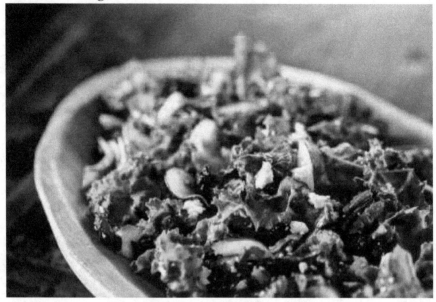

Creamy Mushroom Grits

Prep:

10 mins

Cook:

45 mins

Additional:

8 hrs 30 mins

Total:

9 hrs 25 mins

Servings:

4

Yield:

4 large servings

Ingredients

1 cup stone-ground white corn grits

½ cup shredded Parmesan cheese

4 dried morel mushrooms, or more to taste

3 cups whole milk

3 cups vegetarian chicken-flavored broth

Directions

1

Place grits in a bowl with water to cover. Set aside to soak, 8 hours to overnight. Skim any debris that floats to top, rinse well, and drain.

2

Bring broth to a boil in a saucepan; remove from heat. Add mushrooms and soak until soft, about 30 minutes. Strain mushrooms, reserving broth. Chop mushrooms.

3

Bring reserved broth and milk to a boil in saucepan over high heat. Stir grits in gradually, add mushrooms, and decrease heat to low. Cover and cook, stirring occasionally, until grits are soft and creamy, 40 to 50 minutes. Stir in Parmesan cheese until melted.

Nutrition

Per Serving: 310 calories; protein 14.3g; carbohydrates 41.9g; fat 9.3g; cholesterol 27.1mg; sodium 564mg.

Creamy Breakfast Polenta

Servings:

6

Yield:

6 servings

Ingredients

3 ½ cups Silk® Unsweetened Coconutmilk

¼ cup non-dairy cream cheese

Chopped parsley, chives or other herbs, for garnish

1 teaspoon salt

1 cup organic cornmeal

1 tablespoon vegan margarine

Directions

1

Bring Silk and salt to a boil in a medium saucepan. Slowly stir in cornmeal.

2

Return to a boil, then reduce to a simmer and cook for 15 minutes until very thick, stirring often to prevent polenta from sticking to pan.

3

Remove from heat and stir in cream cheese and margarine until fully incorporated.

4

Spoon into a serving dish or press gently into a large oiled bowl, then turn over for molded polenta.

5

Garnish with parsley, chives or other chopped herbs.

Nutrition

Per Serving: 148 calories; protein 2g; carbohydrates 19g; fat 6.5g; sodium 479.5mg.

Georgia Shake

Prep:

5 mins

Total:

5 mins

Servings:

1

Yield:

1 serving

Ingredients

½ cup milk

¾ cup chocolate ice cream

1 chocolate covered peanut butter cup, crumbled

Directions

1

In a blender, combine milk, peanut butter cup and ice cream. Blend until smooth.

Nutrition

Per Serving: 362 calories; protein 9.5g; carbohydrates 43g; fat 18.5g; cholesterol 44.4mg; sodium 178.6mg.

Tofu Smoothie

Prep:

5 mins

Total:

5 mins

Servings:

4

Yield:

4 servings

Ingredients

⅓ (10.75 ounce) package dessert tofu

1 cup orange juice

5 frozen peach slices

1 (8 ounce) container strawberry yogurt

3 frozen strawberries

Directions

1

In a blender, combine tofu, strawberries, peach slices, yogurt and orange juice. Blend until smooth.

Nutrition

Per Serving: 96 calories; protein 3.3g; carbohydrates 19.9g; fat 0.6g; cholesterol 1.2mg; sodium 42.2mg.

Greek Pita Pockets

Prep:

15 mins

Cook:

10 mins

Total:

25 mins

Servings:

4

Yield:

4 servings

Ingredients

½ cup Greek-style (thick) unflavored yogurt

⅔ cup Nikos® feta cheese crumbles

1 lemon, juiced

4 ounces bulk pork sausage

1 small onion, diced

¾ cup wild mushrooms, chopped

1 cup fresh baby spinach leaves, packed

⅓ cup Greek olives, diced

6 eggs, beaten

2 pitas, halved crosswise

Directions

1

In small bowl, stir together yogurt and lemon juice; set aside.

2

In nonstick skillet over medium-high heat, cook sausage, stirring frequently and crumbling for 2 minutes. Add onion, olives, and mushrooms; cook 4 minutes more.

3

Add spinach leaves and cook until wilted and sausage is fully cooked, about 1 to 3 minutes. Add eggs and cook, stirring constantly until almost dry. Remove from heat and stir in feta.

4

Stuff each pita half with feta-egg mixture. Serve immediately with lemon yogurt.

Nutrition

Per Serving: 382 calories; protein 21g; carbohydrates 23.4g; fat 23.4g; cholesterol 317.3mg; sodium 895.8mg.

Veggies Bakes

Prep:

20 mins

Cook:

40 mins

Total:

1 hr

Servings:

4

Yield:

4 servings

Ingredients

2 large red onions, each cut into 8 wedges

2 large carrots, cut into 1/2-inch slices

½ teaspoon ground cumin

½ large rutabaga, peeled and cut into 3/4-inch cubes

½ cup olive oil

3 tablespoons butter, melted

1 ½ teaspoons curry powder

1 ½ large sweet potatoes, cut into 3/4-inch slices, then into thirds

¾ teaspoon ground turmeric

½ teaspoon salt

Directions

1

Preheat oven to 450 degrees F.

2

Combine red onions, carrots, sweet potatoes, and rutabaga in a large bowl. Pour in olive oil and butter. Add curry powder, turmeric, salt, and cumin; toss until thoroughly coated. Transfer to a large baking dish.

3

Bake in the preheated oven, uncovered, until almost tender, 20 to 30 minutes. Toss. Continue baking until vegetables are fork-tender, 20 to 30 minutes more.

Nutrition

Per Serving: 546 calories; protein 5.3g; carbohydrates 53.4g; fat 36.3g; cholesterol 22.9mg; sodium 494.3mg.

Banana Smoothie

Prep:

5 mins

Total:

5 mins

Servings:

1

Yield:

1 servings

Ingredients

1 cup milk

5 (1 gram) packets low calorie granulated sugar substitute (such as Sweet 'n Low®)

1 ½ bananas

Directions

1

Blend milk, bananas, and sugar substitute in a blender or food processor until smooth.

Nutrition

Per Serving: 280 calories; protein 10g; carbohydrates 56.8g; fat 5.4g; cholesterol 19.5mg; sodium 101.8mg.

Blueberry Pancakes

Prep:

20 mins

Cook:

20 mins

Total:

40 mins

Servings:

4

Yield:

4 pancakes

Ingredients

1 cup all-purpose flour
⅛ teaspoon ground nutmeg
⅛ teaspoon ground cinnamon
1 tablespoon white sugar
1 teaspoon baking powder
1 egg
2 tablespoons vegetable oil
¾ cup fresh blueberries
½ cup plain yogurt
½ cup milk

Directions

1

Preheat griddle over medium heat. Stir together the flour, baking powder, nutmeg, cinnamon and sugar, set aside.

2

In a medium bowl, stir together the egg, yogurt, milk and oil. Gradually stir in the flour mixture, then fold in the blueberries.

3

Pour batter onto hot greased griddle, two tablespoons at a time. Cook over medium heat until bubbles pop and stay open, then turn over and cook on the other side until golden.

Nutrition

Per Serving: 255 calories; protein 7.1g; carbohydrates 34.3g; fat 10.1g; cholesterol 52.9mg; sodium 166.9mg.

CHAPTER 2: LUNCH

Quinoa Jambalaya

Prep:

10 mins

Cook:

30 mins

Total:

40 mins

Servings:

6

Yield:

6 servings

Ingredients

1 tablespoon vegetable oil

2 cups chicken broth

1 pound kielbasa (Polish) sausage, halved lengthwise and sliced

6 miniature multi-colored sweet peppers, diced

1 teaspoon dried oregano

1 teaspoon dried thyme

½ sweet onion (such as Vidalia®), diced

¼ teaspoon celery salt

1 pinch red pepper flakes

½ teaspoon cayenne pepper

1 cup quinoa

½ cup marinara sauce

Directions

1

Heat oil in a large skillet over medium heat; cook and stir sausage until browned, about 5 minutes. Add onion to sausage; cook and stir until slightly browned, about 5 minutes. Stir sweet pepper, oregano, thyme, cayenne pepper, celery salt, and red pepper flakes into sausage mixture; cook and stir until fragrant, about 2 minutes.

2

Mix quinoa into sausage mixture; cook and stir until quinoa is slightly toasted, about 1 minute. Pour broth and marinara sauce over quinoa mixture. Cover skillet and simmer until quinoa is tender, about 15-17 minutes.

Nutrition

Per Serving: 420 calories; protein 14.7g; carbohydrates 26.1g; fat 27.8g; cholesterol 56.1mg; sodium 1091mg.

Salad with Shrimps

Prep:

30 mins

Cook:

10 mins

Total:

40 mins

Servings:

4

Yield:

4 servings

Ingredients

1 pound fresh asparagus, trimmed and sliced diagonally into 2-inch pieces

2 teaspoons white sugar

2 cups chopped tomatoes

½ cup diced green bell pepper

¼ cup finely chopped red onion

¼ cup tomato juice

3 tablespoons red wine vinegar

1 tablespoon olive oil

1 pound large peeled and deveined cooked shrimp

2 cups cubed and seeded English cucumber

2 cloves garlic, minced

⅛ teaspoon hot pepper sauce

1 pinch salt and ground black pepper to taste

8 cups mixed salad greens

¼ cup thinly sliced fresh basil

Directions

1

Place a steamer insert into a saucepan and fill with water to just below the bottom of the steamer. Bring water to a boil. Add asparagus, cover, and steam until crisp-tender, about 4 minutes. Drain and rinse in ice cold water; drain well.

2

Combine steamed asparagus, shrimp, cucumber, tomatoes, bell pepper, onion, and basil in a large bowl.

3

Combine tomato juice, vinegar, oil, garlic, sugar, hot sauce, salt, and pepper in a small bowl. Stir dressing with a whisk until well blended. Pour over shrimp mixture and toss well. Divide greens among 4 plates and top each with 2 cups of the shrimp salad.

Nutrition

Per Serving: 226 calories; protein 29.5g; carbohydrates 17.6g; fat 5.3g; cholesterol 221.3mg; sodium 374.1mg.

Thai Steak

Prep:

15 mins

Cook:

10 mins

Total:

25 mins

Servings:

6

Yield:

6 servings

Ingredients

½ teaspoon ground black pepper

¼ teaspoon kosher salt

¼ cup fresh lime juice

2 tablespoons soy sauce

1 tablespoon brown sugar

⅓ cup fresh Thai basil leaves

1 tablespoon fish sauce

1 (1 1/2-pound) flank steak

2 teaspoons minced garlic

2 heads romaine lettuce

⅓ cup fresh mint leaves

⅓ cup fresh cilantro leaves

1 teaspoon chile-garlic sauce (such as Sriracha®)

Directions

1

Preheat an outdoor grill for medium-high heat and lightly oil the grate. Sprinkle pepper and salt onto flank steak.

2

Cook steak on preheated grill until desired doneness is reached, 5 to 6 minutes per side. An instant-read thermometer inserted into the center should read 140 degrees F.

3

Whisk lime juice, soy sauce, brown sugar, fish sauce, garlic, and chile-garlic sauce together in a bowl.

4

Mix romaine lettuce, mint, cilantro, and basil together in a bowl; spoon about 6 tablespoons lime juice mixture over romaine mixture. Toss to coat.

5

Cut steak into strips and place strips into remaining lime juice mixture; let sit for steak to marinate, approximately 2 minutes. Place steak on romaine mixture.

Nutrition

Per Serving: 132 calories; protein 15.7g; carbohydrates 8g; fat 4.5g; cholesterol 26.9mg; sodium 639.5mg.

Beef Soup

Prep:

10 mins

Cook:

50 mins

Total:

1 hr

Servings:

8

Yield:

8 servings

Ingredients

1 pound ground beef
2 quarts water
1 (16 ounce) package frozen mixed vegetables
1 onion, chopped
4 potatoes, peeled and cubed
8 cubes beef bouillon, crumbled
½ teaspoon ground black pepper
1 (14.5 ounce) can diced tomatoes

Directions

1

In a large pot over medium heat, cook beef until brown; drain.

2

In a large pot over medium heat, combine cooked beef, water, tomatoes, onion, potatoes, mixed vegetables, bouillon and pepper. Bring to a boil, then reduce heat and simmer 45 minutes.

Nutrition

Per Serving: 254 calories; protein 14.6g; carbohydrates 30.5g; fat 8.3g; cholesterol 34.4mg; sodium 1014.1mg.

Beef Saute

Prep:

20 mins

Cook:

45 mins

Total:

1 hr 5 mins

Servings:

4

Yield:

4 servings

Ingredients

9 fluid ounces red wine

1 onion, chopped

1 sprig fresh thyme

2 tablespoons butter

1 ½ pounds beef skirt steak, cut into cubes

2 cloves garlic, chopped

1 tablespoon all-purpose flour

salt and pepper to taste

9 ounces mixed wild mushrooms

1 cup beef stock

Directions

1

In a skillet over medium heat, combine red wine, onion, garlic, and thyme. Bring to a boil, and cook until volume is reduced by about 1/4. Set aside, and allow to cool.

2

Melt butter in a skillet over medium heat until just beginning to brown.
Add beef, and cook until evenly brown. Remove beef, and stir into
cooled wine mixture. Set aside while preparing sauce.

3

Sprinkle flour into skillet. Reduce heat, and cook slowly until flour is
browned. Gradually stir in beef stock, and stir until mixture comes to a
boil. Season with salt and pepper, and simmer uncovered for about 10
minutes.

4

Stir in beef and wine mixture. Cover, and cook very gently for 40 to 45
minutes. Lay mushrooms on top of beef. Cover, and simmer for about
10 more minutes. Transfer beef and mushrooms to a serving dish.
Taste sauce, and adjust seasonings. Simmer until sauce has reduced to
desired consistency, then pour over meat.

Nutrition

Per Serving: 433 calories; protein 39.8g; carbohydrates 9.2g; fat 20.4g;
cholesterol 85.1mg; sodium 452.6mg.

Tabbouleh Salad

Prep:

20 mins

Additional:

15 mins

Total:

35 mins

Servings:

8

Yield:

8 servings

Ingredients

3 cups chopped flat-leaf parsley
2 cups finely chopped pineapple
2 cups pomegranate seeds
½ cup fresh lemon juice
½ cup minced onion
¼ cup minced fresh mint leaves
⅔ cup olive oil
salt and ground black pepper to taste
2 cups finely chopped small cucumber

Directions

1

Mix parsley, cucumber, pineapple, pomegranate seeds, onion, and mint in a large bowl. Drizzle olive oil and lemon juice over the salad and toss to coat; season with salt and pepper.

2

Refrigerate salad until chilled, at least 15 minutes.

Nutrition

Per Serving: 231 calories; protein 1.7g; carbohydrates 17.8g; fat 18.4g; sodium 35.3mg.

Scalloped Scallops

Prep:

10 mins

Cook:

20 mins

Total:

30 mins

Servings:

4

Yield:

4 servings

Ingredients

5 tablespoons butter, divided

salt and ground black pepper to taste

1 pound sea scallops

1 cup half-and-half

¾ cup milk

½ cup bread crumbs

3 tablespoons all-purpose flour

Directions

1

Preheat oven to 400 degrees F. Butter an 8-inch square baking dish.

2

Melt 3 tablespoons butter in a saucepan over medium heat. Cook and stir scallops in melted butter until lightly browned, about 5 minutes. Stir flour into scallop mixture until dissolved, 2 to 3 minutes.

3

Gradually pour half-and-half and milk into scallop mixture, while stirring constantly until milk mixture is thickened, 6 to 10 minutes; season with salt and pepper. Pour scallop mixture into the prepared baking dish.

4

Place remaining 2 tablespoons butter in microwave-safe bowl and heat in microwave until melted, 10-20 seconds. Stir bread crumbs into melted butter until coated; sprinkle over scallop mixture.

5

Bake in the preheated oven until bread crumbs are browned, about 10 minutes.

Nutrition

Per Serving: 451 calories; protein 34.3g; carbohydrates 24.2g; fat 24.1g; cholesterol 132.7mg; sodium 610.1mg.

Hoisin Pork

Prep:

30 mins

Cook:

20 mins

Total:

50 mins

Servings:

4

Yield:

4 servings

Ingredients

1 pound boneless pork chops, cut into stir-fry strips

1 tablespoon hoisin sauce

1 tablespoon cornstarch

2 tablespoons hoisin sauce

1 tablespoon white sugar

1 teaspoon red pepper flakes, or to taste

1 tablespoon sesame oil

2 cloves garlic, minced

¼ cup chicken broth

2 teaspoons minced fresh ginger root

1 tablespoon cornstarch

1 tablespoon rice vinegar

1 carrot, peeled and sliced

1 (4 ounce) can sliced water chestnuts, drained

2 green onions, sliced

1 green bell pepper, sliced

Directions

1

Mix the sliced pork, 1 tablespoon hoisin sauce, and 1 tablespoon cornstarch together in a bowl. Set aside. Combine the remaining 2 tablespoons hoisin sauce, chicken broth, and 1 tablespoon cornstarch with rice vinegar, sugar, and cayenne pepper in small bowl. Set aside.

2

Heat the sesame oil in a skillet over medium-high heat. Stir in the pork; cook and stir until the pork begins to brown, about 5 minutes. Add the garlic and ginger; cook and stir until fragrant. Mix in the carrot, bell pepper, and water chestnuts, cooking until the carrots are tender. Stir in the reserved hoisin sauce mixture and continue cooking and stirring until the flavors are combined, about 3 minutes.

Nutrition

Per Serving: 235 calories; protein 15.6g; carbohydrates 17.5g; fat 11.4g; cholesterol 39.3mg; sodium 295.2mg.

Apple Chicken

Prep:

10 mins

Cook:

20 mins

Total:

30 mins

Servings:

4

Yield:

4 servings

Ingredients

1 link Apple Chicken Sausage, sliced

1 quart fresh strawberries, hulled and quartered

1 medium Granny Smith apple, cored and cut into chunks

2 tablespoons honey

⅓ cup walnut pieces, toasted

¼ cup crumbled low-fat feta cheese

1 (5 ounce) package pre-washed spring mixed greens

2 tablespoons cider vinegar

1 tablespoon canola oil

Directions

1

In a non-stick skillet, over medium heat, lightly brown sausage. Set aside. In a large salad bowl, combine salad greens, strawberries, apple, walnuts, cheese and sausage.

2

In a small bowl, combine vinegar, honey and oil. Pour over salad and toss. Serve.

Nutrition

Per Serving: 272 calories; protein 7.9g; carbohydrates 29.5g; fat 15.6g; cholesterol 23.3mg; sodium 321.6mg.

Cranberry Pork

Prep:

25 mins

Cook:

45 mins

Total:

1 hr 10 mins

Servings:

6

Yield:

6 servings

Ingredients

6 pork chops
¼ teaspoon ground black pepper
2 cups fresh or frozen cranberries
1 teaspoon salt
water as needed
¾ cup white sugar

Directions

1

In a skillet, brown chops slowly in oil; drain.

2

Add cranberries, sugar, salt and pepper to chops with 1/2 cup water to start. Bring to boil; reduce heat. Simmer, covered, for about 45 minutes or until tender but not dry. Add water if necessary to keep chops from drying out.

Nutrition

Per Serving: 229 calories; protein 13.9g; carbohydrates 29.5g; fat 6.3g; cholesterol 37.1mg; sodium 409.1mg.

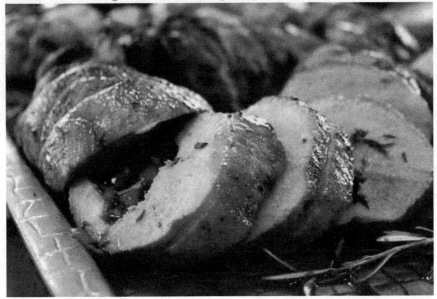

Chicken with Wild Rice Soup

Prep:

20 mins

Cook:

1 hr 55 mins

Total:

2 hrs 15 mins

Servings:

8

Yield:

8 servings

Ingredients

1 ⅓ cups wild rice

7 cups water

2 tablespoons chicken bouillon granules

1 cup chopped celery

1 cup chopped onion

2 tablespoons vegetable oil

1 cup fresh mushrooms, sliced

¾ cup white wine

¾ teaspoon ground white pepper

½ teaspoon salt

½ cup margarine

¾ cup all-purpose flour

1 (3 pound) whole chicken, cut into pieces

4 cups milk

Directions

1

Cook the wild rice according to package directions, but remove from heat about 15 minutes before it's done. Drain the excess liquid, and set aside.

2

In a stock pot over high heat, combine the chicken and the water. Bring to a boil, and then reduce heat to low. Simmer for 40 minutes, or until chicken is cooked and tender. Remove chicken from the pot, and allow it to cool. Strain the broth from the pot, and reserve for later. When chicken is cool, remove the meat from the bones, cut into bite size pieces, and reserve. Discard the fat and the bones.

3

In the same stock pot over medium heat, saute the celery and onion in the oil for 5 minutes. Add the mushrooms, and cover. Cook for 5 to 10 minutes, stirring occasionally, until everything is tender. Return the broth to the stock pot, and add the partially cooked wild rice. Stir in the bouillon, white pepper and salt; simmer, uncovered, for 15 minutes.

4

Meanwhile, melt margarine in a medium saucepan over medium heat. Stir in the flour until smooth. Whisk in the milk, and continue cooking until mixture is bubbly and thick. Add some of the broth mixture to the milk mixture, continuing to stir, then stir all of the milk mixture into the broth mixture.

5

Mix in the reserved chicken meat and the white wine. Allow this to heat through for about 15 minutes.

Nutrition

Per Serving: 572 calories; protein 33.6g; carbohydrates 38.1g; fat 29.6g; cholesterol 84.5mg; sodium 431.7mg.

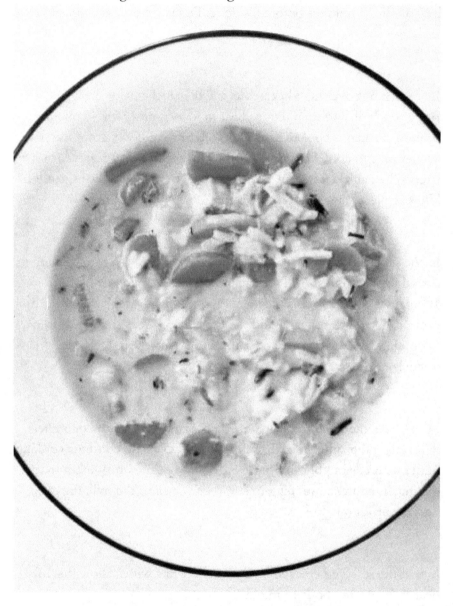

Lentil Soup

Prep:

20 mins

Cook:

6 hrs

Total:

6 hrs 20 mins

Servings:

10

Yield:

10 servings

Ingredients

7 cups water

1 pound cooked, smoked lean ham, cut into chunks

½ teaspoon dried thyme

1 (14.5 ounce) can low-sodium diced tomatoes, undrained

6 ounces sliced carrots

1 ¾ cups dried lentils, rinsed

8 ounces chopped onion

6 ounces chopped celery

5 cloves garlic, minced

½ teaspoon ground black pepper

1 bay leaf

Directions

1

Combine water, ham, tomatoes, lentils, onion, carrots, celery, garlic, pepper, salt, thyme, and bay leaf in a slow cooker.

2

Cover and cook on low until lentils and vegetables are as soft as you like, 6 to 8 hours. Remove bay leaf before serving.

Nutrition

Per Serving: 259 calories; protein 18g; carbohydrates 26.7g; fat 8.9g; cholesterol 25.4mg; sodium 736.5mg.

Tomato Bean Soup

Prep:

15 mins

Cook:

30 mins

Total:

45 mins

Servings:

4

Yield:

4 servings

Ingredients

1 (15 ounce) can black beans, undrained

1 cup low-sodium chicken broth

cooking spray

1 (15 ounce) can black beans, undrained

1 small onion, chopped

2 teaspoons ground cumin

1 teaspoon minced garlic

1 (10 ounce) can diced tomatoes with green chile peppers (such as RO*TEL®)

4 teaspoons lime juice

2 tablespoons chopped fresh cilantro

Directions

1

Place 1 can black beans and chicken broth into a blender. Cover and puree until smooth.

2

Heat a large saucepan coated with cooking spray over medium-high heat; cook and stir onion and garlic until onion is tender, about 5 minutes. Stir remaining 1 can black beans and liquid, tomatoes, yogurt, lime juice, cumin, red pepper flakes, and pureed beans into onion mixture; bring to a boil. Reduce heat to low, cover, and simmer for 25 to 30 minutes, stirring occasionally. Garnish with cilantro to serve.

Nutrition

Per Serving: 237 calories; protein 15.7g; carbohydrates 42.3g; fat 1.5g; cholesterol 2.2mg; sodium 1142.6mg.

Onion Tilapia

Prep:

10 mins

Cook:

15 mins

Additional:

2 mins

Total:

27 mins

Servings:

1

Yield:

1 tilapia fillet

Ingredients

¼ large lemon

1 (6 ounce) tilapia fillet, patted dry

1 tablespoon grated fresh Parmesan cheese

¼ large red onion, coarsely chopped

1 teaspoon minced garlic

1 teaspoon butter, divided

salt and ground black pepper to taste

1 tablespoon extra-virgin olive oil

Directions

1

Squeeze lemon juice over tilapia; season lightly with salt and black pepper.

2

Heat olive oil in a nonstick skillet over medium heat. Melt 1/2 teaspoon butter in hot oil. Add chopped onion and minced garlic; cook and stir until onion begins to look translucent, about 5 minutes.

3

Reduce heat to medium-low. Push onion mixture to sides of the skillet. Melt remaining 1/2 teaspoon of butter in the skillet. Place tilapia in the center of the skillet and cover with onion mixture. Cover skillet and cook tilapia until it starts to turn golden, about 5 minutes. Push onion mixture to the sides again and flip tilapia. Cover and cook until second side is golden and flakes easily with a fork, about 6 minutes more.

4

Remove skillet from heat. Top tilapia with grated Parmesan cheese, cover, and let stand until cheese is melted, about 3 minutes.

Nutrition

Per Serving: 371 calories; protein 37.3g; carbohydrates 7.6g; fat 21.4g; cholesterol 76.7mg; sodium 337.8mg.

Pork Loin

Prep:
15 mins
Cook:
1 hr 5 mins
Additional:
8 hrs
Total:
9 hrs 20 mins
Servings:
6
Yield:
1 pork roast

Ingredients

1 quart cold water
¼ cup salt
⅓ cup maple syrup
2 tablespoons maple syrup
3 cloves garlic, crushed
1 tablespoon cracked black pepper
½ teaspoon red pepper flakes
3 tablespoons chopped fresh ginger
1 (2 1/2 pound) boneless pork loin roast
salt and freshly ground black pepper
2 teaspoons dried rosemary
1 tablespoon vegetable oil
2 tablespoons Dijon mustard

Directions

1

Mix water, salt, 1/3 cup maple syrup, garlic, ginger, rosemary, black pepper, and red pepper flakes in a large bowl. Place pork loin in brine mixture and refrigerate for 8 to 10 hours.

2

Remove pork from brine, pat dry, and season all sides with salt and black pepper.

3

Preheat oven to 325 degrees F.

4

Heat vegetable oil in an oven-proof skillet over high heat. Cook pork, turning to brown each side, about 10 minutes total.

5

Transfer skillet to the oven and roast until pork is browned, about 40 minutes.

6

Mix 2 tablespoons maple syrup and Dijon mustard together in a small bowl.

7

Remove pork roast from the oven and spread maple syrup mixture on all sides. Cook for an additional 15 minutes, until the pork is no longer pink in the center. An instant-read thermometer inserted into the center should read 145 degrees F.

Nutrition

Per Serving: 376 calories; protein 30.7g; carbohydrates 19.3g; fat 18.9g; cholesterol 92mg; sodium 225.3mg.

Juicy Chicken

Prep:

20 mins

Cook:

10 mins

Total:

30 mins

Servings:

5

Yield:

5 servings

Ingredients

½ cup soy sauce

1 pound skinless, boneless chicken breast halves - cut into 2 inch pieces

½ cup sherry or white cooking wine

¼ teaspoon ground ginger

1 pinch garlic powder

1 bunch green onions, chopped

½ cup chicken broth

Directions

1

In a small saucepan, combine the soy sauce, sherry, chicken broth, ginger, garlic powder and green onions. Bring to a boil, and immediately remove from heat. Set aside.

2

Preheat your oven's broiler. Thread chicken pieces onto metal or bamboo skewers. Arrange on a broiler pan that has been coated with cooking spray. Spoon 1 or 2 tablespoons of the sauce over each chicken skewer.

3

Place the pan under the broiler, and broil for about 3 minutes, until browned. Remove from the oven, turn over, and spoon more sauce onto each one. Return to the oven until chicken is cooked through and nicely browned.

Nutrition

Per Serving: 152 calories; protein 23.5g; carbohydrates 9.2g; fat 1.2g; cholesterol 52.7mg; sodium 1652.9mg.

Green Beans with Shallots and Prosciutto

Prep:

5 mins

Cook:

10 mins

Total:

15 mins

Servings:

4

Yield:

4 servings

Ingredients

3 tablespoons unsalted butter, divided
2 ounces prosciutto, chopped
1 pound haricots verts (thin French green beans)
2 tablespoons water
2 shallots, thinly sliced
½ teaspoon salt

Directions

1

Melt 1 tablespoon butter in a large skillet over medium-high heat. Add shallots and prosciutto; cook until prosciutto begins to crisp, 3 to 4 minutes. Remove mixture to a plate and set aside.

2

Add remaining butter to the skillet and add haricots verts. Saute for 1 to 2 minutes, then add water and cover. Let green beans steam until most of the water is absorbed, about 5 minutes. Season with salt.

3

Remove green beans to a nice serving dish; top with the shallots and prosciutto.

Nutrition

Per Serving: 182 calories; protein 5.5g; carbohydrates 12.3g; fat 13.3g; cholesterol 35.4mg; sodium 576.2mg.

Paella

Prep:

30 mins

Cook:

30 mins

Total:

1 hr

Servings:

8

Yield:

8 servings

Ingredients

2 tablespoons olive oil

1 tablespoon paprika

2 pounds skinless, boneless chicken breasts, cut into 2 inch pieces

2 tablespoons olive oil, divided

3 cloves garlic, crushed

2 teaspoons dried oregano

1 teaspoon crushed red pepper flakes

1 pinch saffron threads

salt and black pepper to taste

1 bay leaf

1 quart chicken stock

2 lemons, zested

2 tablespoons olive oil

½ bunch Italian flat leaf parsley, chopped

1 Spanish onion, chopped

1 red bell pepper, coarsely chopped

1 pound chorizo sausage, casings removed and crumbled

2 cups uncooked short-grain white rice
1 pound shrimp, peeled and deveined

Directions

1

In a medium bowl, mix together 2 tablespoons olive oil, paprika, oregano, and salt and pepper. Stir in chicken pieces to coat. Cover, and refrigerate.

2

Heat 2 tablespoons olive oil in a large skillet or paella pan over medium heat. Stir in garlic, red pepper flakes, and rice. Cook, stirring, to coat rice with oil, about 3 minutes. Stir in saffron threads, bay leaf, parsley, chicken stock, and lemon zest. Bring to a boil, cover, and reduce heat to medium low. Simmer 20 minutes.

3

Meanwhile, heat 2 tablespoons olive oil in a separate skillet over medium heat. Stir in marinated chicken and onion; cook 5 minutes. Stir in bell pepper and sausage; cook 5 minutes. Stir in shrimp; cook, turning the shrimp, until both sides are pink.

4

Spread rice mixture onto a serving tray. Top with meat and seafood mixture.

Nutrition

Per Serving: 736 calories; protein 55.7g; carbohydrates 45.7g; fat 35.1g; cholesterol 202.5mg; sodium 1204.2mg.

Yogurt Soup

Prep:

10 mins

Cook:

25 mins

Total:

35 mins

Servings:

4

Yield:

4 servings

Ingredients

4 cups whole milk

3 cups plain yogurt

5 tablespoons all-purpose flour

2 cups water

2 egg yolks

4 teaspoons chicken bouillon granules

1 teaspoon salt

½ teaspoon ground black pepper

2 tablespoons lemon juice

Directions

1

Beat milk, yogurt, egg yolks, and all-purpose flour in a large bowl with an electric mixer.

2

Meanwhile, bring water and chicken bouillon to a boil in a large soup pot. Reduce heat to medium-low and add yogurt mixture, lemon juice, salt, and pepper, stirring occasionally until mixture thickens, about 20 minutes.

Nutrition

Per Serving: 332 calories; protein 20.2g; carbohydrates 32.9g; fat 13.4g; cholesterol 138.1mg; sodium 1187.2mg.

Tofu Turkey

Servings:

10

Yield:

10 servings

Ingredients

5 (16 ounce) packages extra-firm tofu

½ teaspoon orange zest

2 tablespoons sesame oil

1 cup chopped mushrooms

1 red onion, finely diced

1 ⅓ cups diced celery

2 cloves garlic, minced

⅛ cup dried sage

2 teaspoons dried thyme

salt and pepper to taste

1 ½ teaspoons dried rosemary

¼ cup tamari

¼ cup tamari

2 tablespoons miso paste

5 tablespoons orange juice

3 cups prepared herb stuffing

½ cup sesame oil

1 teaspoon honey mustard

3 sprigs fresh rosemary

Directions

1

Line a medium sized, round colander with a cheese cloth or a clean dish towel. Place the crumbled tofu in the colander. Place another cheese cloth over the top of the tofu. Place the colander over the top of a bowl to catch the liquid. Place a heavy weight on top of tofu. Refrigerate the colander, tofu and weight for 2 to 3 hours.

2

Make the stuffing: In a large frying pan saute onion, celery and mushrooms in 2 tablespoons of the sesame oil until tender. Add the garlic, sage, thyme, salt and pepper, rosemary and 1/4 cup of the tamari. Stir well; cook for 5 minutes. Add prepared herb stuffing and mix well. Remove from heat.

3

Preheat the oven to 400 degrees F. Grease a cookie sheet.

4

Combine 1/2 cup sesame oil, 1/4 cup tamari, miso, orange juice, mustard and orange zest in a small bowl; mix well.

5

Remove the weight from the tofu. Hollow out the tofu so that there is one inch of tofu still lining the colander. Place the scooped out tofu in a separate bowl. Brush the tofu lining with a small amount of the miso seasoning. Scoop the stuffing into the center of the tofu shell. Place the leftover tofu on top of the stuffing and press down firmly. Turn the stuffed tofu onto the prepared cookie sheet. Putting the leftover tofu side of the "turkey" (the flat side) down. Gently press on the sides of the "turkey" to form a more oval shape. Brush the tofu turkey with 1/2 of the oil-tamari mixture. Place the sprigs of rosemary on top of the tofu. Cover the "turkey" with foil.

6

Bake for one hour. After one hour, remove "turkey" from the oven and remove the foil. Baste the "turkey" with the remaining tamari-oil sauce (reserving 4 tablespoons of sauce). Return "turkey" to oven and bake another hour or until the tofu turkey is golden brown. Place the tofu turkey on a serving platter, brush with the remaining tamari-oil mixture and serve hot.

Nutrition

Per Serving: 470 calories; protein 26.7g; carbohydrates 22.4g; fat 32.4g; sodium 1294.9mg.

Celeriac Salad

Prep:

15 mins

Cook:

30 mins

Total:

45 mins

Servings:

12

Yield:

6 cups

Ingredients

1 celeriac (celery root), peeled and cut into 1/2-inch pieces

⅓ cup heavy cream

3 tablespoons butter

3 potatoes, peeled and cut into 1/2-inch pieces

Directions

1

Place the celeriac cubes into a large pot and cover with salted water. Bring to a boil over high heat, then reduce heat to medium-low, cover, and simmer 12 minutes. Add the potatoes, and continue boiling until the vegetables are very tender, about 15 minutes more. Drain and allow to steam dry for a minute or two.

2

Return the vegetables to the pot, and stir over medium-high heat until liquid is no longer pooling from the vegetables. Remove from the heat, and pour in the cream and butter. Mash with a potato masher until almost smooth.

Nutrition

Per Serving: 117 calories; protein 2.2g; carbohydrates 15.6g; fat 5.6g; cholesterol 16.7mg; sodium 92.8mg.

Avocado Salad

Servings:

2

Yield:

2 servings

Ingredients

2 medium avocados
1 pinch chili powder
2 small tomatoes, chopped
1 tablespoon chopped fresh cilantro, or to taste
½ tablespoon ground black pepper
1 (5 ounce) can light tuna (such as Century®)
salt to taste

Directions

1

Scoop out avocado contents and place in a bowl. Set aside shells.

2

Mix in tuna, tomatoes, cilantro, pepper, chili powder, and salt. Divide mixture between shells to serve.

Nutrition

Per Serving: 417 calories; protein 21.1g; carbohydrates 22g; fat 30.3g; cholesterol 18.9mg; sodium 133.6mg.

Lime Calamari

Prep:

15 mins

Cook:

5 mins

Total:

20 mins

Servings:

10

Yield:

10 appetizer servings

Ingredients

3 cups vegetable oil

1 lemon - cut into wedges, for garnish

1 teaspoon salt

1 teaspoon dried oregano

½ teaspoon ground black pepper

12 squid, cleaned and sliced into rings

¼ cup all-purpose flour

Directions

1

Preheat oil in a heavy, deep frying pan or pot. Oil should be heated to 365 degrees F.

2

In a medium size mixing bowl mix together flour, salt, oregano and black pepper. Dredge squid through flour and spice mixture.

3

Place squid in oil for 2 to 3 minutes or until light brown. Beware of overcooking, squid will be tough if overcooked. Dry squid on paper towels. Serve with wedges of lemon.

Nutrition

Per Serving: 642 calories; protein 8g; carbohydrates 5.2g; fat 66.7g; cholesterol 111.8mg; sodium 254.1mg.

Tofu Parmigiana

Prep:

25 mins

Cook:

20 mins

Total:

45 mins

Servings:

4

Yield:

4 servings

Ingredients

½ cup seasoned bread crumbs

5 tablespoons grated Parmesan cheese

salt to taste

ground black pepper to taste

1 (12 ounce) package firm tofu

2 tablespoons olive oil

2 teaspoons dried oregano, divided

1 (8 ounce) can tomato sauce

1 clove garlic, minced

4 ounces shredded mozzarella cheese

½ teaspoon dried basil

Directions

1

In a small bowl, combine bread crumbs, 2 tablespoons Parmesan cheese, 1 teaspoon oregano, salt, and black pepper.

2

Slice tofu into 1/4 inch thick slices, and place in bowl of cold water. One at a time, press tofu slices into crumb mixture, turning to coat all sides.

3

Heat oil in a medium skillet over medium heat. Cook tofu slices until crisp on one side. Drizzle with a bit more olive oil, turn, and brown on the other side.

4

Combine tomato sauce, basil, garlic, and remaining oregano. Place a thin layer of sauce in an 8 inch square baking pan. Arrange tofu slices in the pan. Spoon remaining sauce over tofu. Top with shredded mozzarella and remaining 3 tablespoons Parmesan.

5

Bake at 400 degrees F for 20-22 minutes.

Nutrition

Per Serving: 357 calories; protein 25.7g; carbohydrates 18.8g; fat 21.5g; cholesterol 23.8mg; sodium 840.7mg.

Garlic Soup

Prep:

15 mins

Cook:

20 mins

Total:

35 mins

Servings:

4

Yield:

4 servings

Ingredients

2 tablespoons olive oil

6 cups chicken stock

2 carrots, cut into matchsticks

1 head garlic, peeled and lightly crushed

salt and pepper to taste

1 red bell pepper, thinly sliced

Directions

1

Heat oil in a large saucepan over medium heat. Stir in garlic and cook until lightly browned, about 5 minutes. Pour in 1 cup of chicken stock, cover, and allow to simmer until the garlic is soft, about 10 minutes.

2

Mash the garlic with a fork into a coarse paste. Pour in remaining chicken stock, increase heat to medium-high, and bring to a boil. Stir in carrots and cook for 1 minute, then add red pepper and continue cooking until vegetables are tender. Season to taste with salt and pepper before serving.

Nutrition

Per Serving: 118 calories; protein 2.4g; carbohydrates 10.9g; fat 7.9g; cholesterol 1.1mg; sodium 1053.2mg.

Sirloin Soup

Prep:

15 mins

Cook:

15 mins

Total:

30 mins

Servings:

8

Yield:

8 servings

Ingredients

2 tablespoons olive oil

2 pounds top sirloin steak, sliced

½ cup red wine

2 cups chunky pasta sauce

2 cloves garlic, minced

1 onion, thinly sliced

Directions

1

Heat the oil in a 10 inch skillet over medium high heat. Add the onions and saute until tender, about 5 minutes. Add the steak strips, turning so that all sides get browned, about 12 minutes.

2

Add the tomato sauce, garlic and red wine. Reduce heat to low and simmer for 10 to 15 minutes, or until the steak is cooked through.

Nutrition

Per Serving: 276 calories; protein 20g; carbohydrates 10.5g; fat 15.4g; cholesterol 61.7mg; sodium 299.9mg.

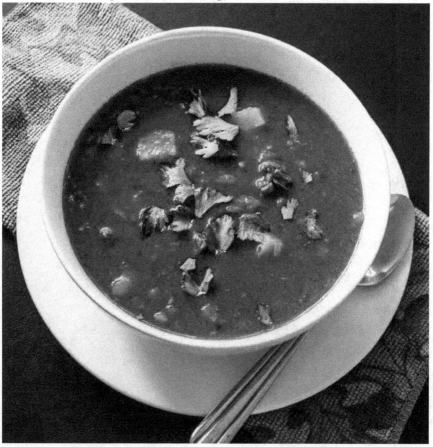

Red Pepper & Goat Cheese Frittata

Prep:

15 mins

Cook:

20 mins

Total:

35 mins

Servings:

4

Yield:

4 servings

Ingredients

2 tablespoons olive oil

1 cup diced roasted red peppers

2 tablespoons minced garlic

½ teaspoon minced fresh basil

⅓ cup heavy cream

salt and pepper to taste

6 small red potatoes, thinly sliced

½ cup crumbled goat cheese

6 eggs

Directions

1

Preheat the oven's broiler and set the oven rack about 6 inches from the heat source.

2

Heat the olive oil in a cast-iron skillet over medium heat, and spread the potatoes into the hot pan in an even layer. Cover the skillet, and cook the potatoes until they start to turn tender, about 10 minutes. Stir in the red peppers and garlic, and sprinkle with salt and pepper. Cook and stir the potato mixture until the garlic begins to soften, about 2 minutes, sprinkle on the basil, and cook the mixture, stirring occasionally, until the basil is cooked, about 2 more minutes.

3

Whisk the eggs and cream together in a bowl, and pour the egg mixture over the vegetables in the skillet. Sprinkle the top with goat cheese, cover the skillet, and reduce the heat to low. Cook until the eggs are set but not dry, 3 to 5 minutes. Uncover the skillet, and place it under the broiler until the top of the frittata has browned, about 2 minutes.

Nutrition

Per Serving: 501 calories; protein 19.4g; carbohydrates 46.3g; fat 27.5g; cholesterol 320mg; sodium 412.9mg.

Sunshine Toast

Prep:

5 mins

Cook:

10 mins

Total:

15 mins

Servings:

1

Yield:

1 serving

Ingredients

1 egg

salt to taste

1 slice bread

2 tablespoons butter, divided

Directions

1

Melt 1 tablespoon butter in a small skillet over medium heat.

2

Using a glass or cookie cutter, create a hole in the middle of the bread, removing the center so it is perfectly circular. Butter the bread lightly on both sides and lightly fry it on one side, and then turn it over. Crack the egg into the hole in the middle of the bread and fry quickly. Be careful that the bread does not burn. Serve warm.

Nutrition

Per Serving: 342 calories; protein 8.4g; carbohydrates 13.1g; fat 28.8g; cholesterol 247.1mg; sodium 403.8mg

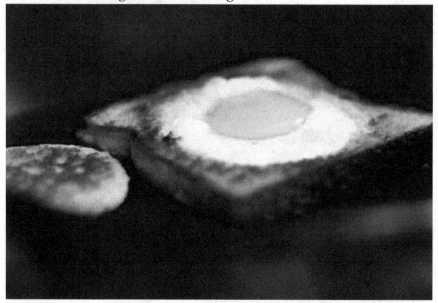

Salmon Salad

Prep:

20 mins

Total:

20 mins

Servings:

6

Yield:

6 servings

Ingredients

2 cups mayonnaise

1 (3 ounce) package smoked salmon, flaked

½ lemon, juiced

2 tablespoons chopped capers

2 Granny Smith apples, cored and sliced

1 ½ cups sweet corn

3 tablespoons chopped fresh dill

Directions

1

Mix mayonnaise, lemon juice, dill, and capers together in a large bowl until smooth. Add apples, corn, and smoked salmon; toss gently until evenly coated. Chill before serving.

Nutrition

Per Serving: 603 calories; protein 4.9g; carbohydrates 17.8g; fat 59.2g; cholesterol 31.1mg; sodium 615.7mg.

Cider Pork Cheeks

Servings:

4

Yield:

4 servings

Ingredients

8 (4 ounce) pork cheeks
salt and freshly ground black pepper to taste
2 tablespoons clarified butter
2 tablespoons apple cider vinegar
2 cups hard apple cider
½ cup all-purpose flour for dredging
1 rib celery, diced
2 cups homemade or low-sodium chicken broth
1 teaspoon finely chopped fresh sage leaves
1 small yellow onion, diced
1 small carrot, diced
1 teaspoon finely chopped fresh rosemary leaves

Directions

1

Season both sides of pork cheeks with salt and pepper. Sprinkle with flour and press it into the meat to coat thoroughly.

2

Heat clarified butter in a pan over medium-high heat. Sear meat on both sides until richly browned, adjusting heat lower if necessary. When cheeks are browned, reduce heat to medium. Transfer cheeks to a plate to rest.

3

Remove all but 2 tablespoons fat from the skillet. Add onions, carrots, and celery to skillet. Cook and stir until softened and sweet, seasoning with a pinch of salt. Add vinegar and stir to deglaze the pan. Pour in the cider and chicken stock. Bring to a simmer. Add sage and rosemary. Reduce heat to low and transfer cheeks back to pan. Cover. Cook until fork tender but not falling apart, 2 to 3 hours depending on the size of the pork cheeks. Transfer to a plate.

4

Bring liquid to a boil over high heat, skimming off fat as it rises to the surface. Reduce volume of liquid by about 60 to 70%. Sauce will start to thicken up. Taste for salt and season as needed. Transfer cheeks back to liquid. Continue to cook over medium-low heat until cheeks are heated through and tender and sauce is thick enough to coat cheeks.

Nutrition

Per Serving: 1619 calories; protein 19.7g; carbohydrates 23.5g; fat 153.3g; cholesterol 193.3mg; sodium 296.7mg.

CHAPTER 3: DINNER

Pork Chops with Black Beans

Prep:

5 mins

Cook:

25 mins

Total:

30 mins

Servings:

4

Yield:

4 servings

Ingredients

4 bone-in pork chops
1 tablespoon chopped fresh cilantro
ground black pepper to taste
1 (15 ounce) can black beans, with liquid
1 cup salsa
1 tablespoon olive oil

Directions

1

Season pork chops with pepper.

2

Heat oil in a large skillet over medium-high heat. Cook pork chops in hot oil until browned, 3 to 5 minutes per side.

3

Pour beans and salsa over pork chops and season with cilantro. Bring to a boil, reduce heat to medium-low, cover the skillet, and simmer until pork chops are cooked no longer pink in the center, 20 to 40 minutes. An instant-read thermometer inserted into the center should read 145 degrees F.

Nutrition

Per Serving: 392 calories; protein 33.8g; carbohydrates 21.8g; fat 18.7g; cholesterol 72.1mg; sodium 836.5mg.

Potato Salad

Prep:

20 mins

Cook:

10 mins

Additional:

6 hrs

Total:

6 hrs 30 mins

Servings:

20

Yield:

20 servings

Ingredients

5 pounds red potatoes, chopped

3 cups mayonnaise

2 cups finely chopped pickles

½ cup chopped red onion

½ cup chopped celery

3 tablespoons prepared mustard

5 hard-cooked eggs, chopped

1 tablespoon apple cider vinegar

½ teaspoon ground black pepper

1 teaspoon salt, or to taste

Directions

1

Place potatoes into a large pot and cover with salted water; bring to a boil. Reduce heat to medium-low and simmer until tender, about 10 minutes. Drain. Return potatoes to empty pot to dry while you mix the dressing. Sprinkle with salt.

2

Stir mayonnaise, pickles, hard-cooked eggs, red onion, celery, mustard, cider vinegar, 1 teaspoon salt, and pepper together in a large bowl. Fold potatoes into the mayonnaise mixture. Allow to chill at least six hours, or overnight, before serving.

Nutrition

Per Serving: 339 calories; protein 4.1g; carbohydrates 20.4g; fat 27.6g; cholesterol 53.5mg; sodium 538.1mg.

Brown Rice Pilaf

Prep:

10 mins

Cook:

55 mins

Total:

1 hr 5 mins

Servings:

2

Yield:

2 servings

Ingredients

½ cup fresh corn kernels

½ cup brown rice

1 ¼ cups chicken broth

½ cup chopped onion

1 tablespoon olive oil

Directions

1

Heat olive oil in a small saucepan over medium heat. Add corn and onion; cook and stir until lightly browned, 5 to 7 minutes. Add rice and stir to coat with oil. Add chicken broth and bring to a boil. Cover and reduce heat to low. Cook until rice is tender, about 45 minutes.

Nutrition

Per Serving: 259 calories; protein 4.8g; carbohydrates 40.7g; fat 8.4g; cholesterol 3.8mg; sodium 730.9mg.

Carrot Pudding

Servings:

7

Yield:

6 to 8 servings

Ingredients

1 cup grated carrots
1 teaspoon baking soda
1 cup peeled and shredded potatoes
1 cup white sugar
1 cup raisins
1 teaspoon ground cinnamon
1 teaspoon ground allspice
1 cup all-purpose flour
1 teaspoon ground cloves
½ cup butter
1 cup white sugar
1 ½ teaspoons vanilla extract
½ cup heavy whipping cream

Directions

1

In a large mixing bowl, combine carrots, potatoes, sugar, raisins, flour, baking soda, ground cinnamon, all spice, and ground cloves. Transfer mixture to a clean 1 pound coffee can. Secure wax paper over the top and place the filled can in a large pot with 2 to 3 inches of water. Cover the pot and bring the water to a simmer.

2

Steam the cake for 2 hours. Serve warm.

3

Buttery sauce: In a medium-size pot, combine butter or margarine, cream, sugar, and vanilla. Heat until the mixture is liquid. Spoon mixture over the warm carrot pudding to serve.

Nutrition

Per Serving: 552 calories; protein 3.6g; carbohydrates 93.8g; fat 19.9g; cholesterol 58.2mg; sodium 295.5mg.

Creamy Polenta with Arrabbiata Sausage Ragout

Prep:

10 mins

Cook:

35 mins

Total:

45 mins

Servings:

4

Yield:

4 servings

Ingredients

Polenta:

2 ½ cups water

2 tablespoons unsalted butter

½ cup milk

1 teaspoon salt

1 cup Italian polenta

½ cup grated Parmigiano-Reggiano cheese

Arrabbiata Sauce and Sausages:

2 tablespoons grapeseed oil or olive oil

2 large bell peppers, seeded and sliced into 1/2-inch thick rings

1 medium sweet onion, cut into 1/2-inch slices

1 (19 ounce) package Italian sausage links

¼ teaspoon crushed red pepper flakes

1 (24 ounce) jar Classico® Tomato and Basil Sauce

Directions

1

In a large saucepan over high heat, bring the water, milk, and salt to a boil. Add the polenta in a slow, steady stream, stirring continuously with a wooden spoon until incorporated.

2

Continue stirring to prevent lumps from forming. Reduce the heat so the mixture bubbles occasionally.

3

Cook, stirring and scraping the bottom and sides of the pan, until the polenta is thick and starts to pull away from the sides of the pan, 35 to 40 minutes.

4

Remove from the heat. Stir in the butter, a few cubes at a time, then stir in the cheese. Keep warm over very low heat.

5

Heat grapeseed oil in a large saute pan over medium heat. Add the sausages and cook following cooking instructions indicated on the packaging, or until no longer pink in the center, about 8 minutes. An instant-read thermometer inserted into the center should read 160 degrees F. Transfer the sausages to a plate.

6

Add the bell peppers and onion to the pan and cook, stirring occasionally, until browned and tender, about 12 minutes.

7

Stir in the pasta sauce and crushed red pepper flakes. Bring to a simmer and return the sausages to the pan. Cover and cook for 10 minutes, then remove from the heat. Slice sausages before serving.

8

To serve, place a mound of polenta onto a plate, and top with the sausage and arrabbiata sauce.

Nutrition

Per Serving: 771 calories; protein 31.7g; carbohydrates 57.9g; fat 46.2g; cholesterol 82.7mg; sodium 2663.4mg.

Manicotti alla Romana

Prep:

1 hr

Cook:

50 mins

Total:

1 hr 50 mins

Servings:

7

Yield:

6 to 8 servings

Ingredients

2 tablespoons olive oil

½ cup chopped onion

6 cloves garlic, finely chopped

1 pound ground beef

salt to taste

2 cups ricotta cheese

2 eggs, beaten

3 cups spaghetti sauce, divided

2 tablespoons butter

2 tablespoons all-purpose flour

1 (10 ounce) package frozen chopped spinach, thawed and drained

1 (12 ounce) package manicotti shells

2 cups half-and-half

¼ cup chopped fresh parsley

1 tablespoon chopped fresh basil

½ cup grated Parmesan cheese

2 tablespoons chicken bouillon granules

Directions

1

Heat oil in a large skillet over medium heat. Saute onions until translucent. Saute garlic for 1 minute and stir in ground beef. Cook until well browned and crumbled. Season with salt and set aside to cool.

2

Cook spinach according to package **Directions**. Meanwhile, bring a large pot of lightly salted water to a boil. Add manicotti shells and parboil for half of the time recommended on the package. Drain and cover with cool water to stop the cooking process and prevent the shells from cracking.

3

To the ground beef mixture add the cooked spinach and ricotta cheese. When the mixture is cool, add the beaten eggs. Spread 1/4 cup spaghetti sauce in the bottom of a 9x13 inch baking dish. Gently drain the manicotti shells and carefully stuff each one with the meat and cheese mixture; place shells in prepared dish. Lightly cover the dish with plastic wrap or a clean, damp towel to prevent shells from cracking.

4

Preheat oven to 350 degrees F.

5

Prepare the white sauce by melting the butter in a small saucepan over medium heat. Stir in flour and chicken bouillon. Increase heat to medium-high and cook, stirring constantly, until it begins to bubble. Stir in half and half and bring to a boil, stirring frequently. Cook for 1 minute, stirring constantly. Remove from heat and stir in parsley. Pour or ladle the sauce evenly over the stuffed shells.

6

Stir the basil into the remaining spaghetti sauce. Carefully pour or ladle spaghetti sauce over the white sauce, trying to layer the sauces without mixing.

7

Cover and bake for 40-45 minutes. Remove from oven, uncover and sprinkle with Parmesan cheese. Bake, uncovered, for 10 minutes more.

Nutrition

Per Serving: 612 calories; protein 27.6g; carbohydrates 58.7g; fat 30.3g; cholesterol 134.2mg; sodium 991.6mg.

Ginger Snapper

Prep:

10 mins

Cook:

20 mins

Total:

30 mins

Servings:

6

Yield:

6 servings

Ingredients

cooking spray
1 cup soy sauce
1 (2 inch) piece fresh ginger root, minced
¼ cup honey
2 cloves garlic, minced
1 (2 pound) whole snapper fillet

Directions

1

Preheat oven to 350 degrees F. Spray a large sheet of aluminum foil with cooking spray.

2

Thoroughly mix the soy sauce, honey, ginger, and garlic in a large bowl. Dip both sides of the fish into the soy sauce mixture, and place onto the aluminum foil. Spoon a little more sauce over the top of the fish. Roll up the aluminum foil to completely enclose the fillet.

3

Bake in the preheated oven until the fish is opaque and flakes easily, about 20 minutes.

Nutrition

Per Serving: 220 calories; protein 33.9g; carbohydrates 15.5g; fat 2.1g; cholesterol 55.5mg; sodium 2474.1mg.

Pantry Puttanesca

Prep:

5 mins

Cook:

16 mins

Total:

21 mins

Servings:

4

Yield:

4 servings

Ingredients

⅓ cup olive oil

¼ cup capers, chopped

3 cloves garlic, minced

¼ teaspoon crushed red pepper flakes

1 teaspoon dried oregano

2 (15 ounce) cans diced tomatoes, drained.

1 (8 ounce) package spaghetti

½ cup chopped pitted kalamata olives

3 anchovy fillets, chopped

Directions

1

Fill a large pot with water. Bring to a rolling boil over high heat.

2

As the water heats, pour the olive oil into a cold skillet and stir in the garlic. Turn heat to medium-low and cook and stir until the garlic is fragrant and begins to turn a golden color, 1 to 2 minutes. Stir in the red pepper flakes, oregano, and anchovies. Cook until anchovies begin to break down, about 2 minutes.

3

Pour tomatoes into skillet, turn heat to medium-high, and bring sauce to a simmer. Use the back of a spoon to break down tomatoes as they cook. Simmer until sauce is reduced and combined, about 12 minutes.

4

Meanwhile, cook the pasta in the boiling water. Drain when still very firm to the bite, about 10 minutes. Reserve 1/2 cup pasta water.

5

Stir the olives and capers into the sauce; add pasta and toss to combine.

6

Toss pasta in sauce until pasta is cooked through and well coated with sauce, about 1 minute. If sauce becomes too thick, stir in some of the reserved pasta water to thin.

Nutrition

Per Serving: 463 calories; protein 10.5g; carbohydrates 53.3g; fat 24g; cholesterol 2.5mg; sodium 944.5mg.

Paprika Tilapia

Prep:

10 mins

Cook:

8 mins

Total:

18 mins

Servings:

4

Yield:

4 servings

Ingredients

3 tablespoons olive oil
½ teaspoon freshly ground black pepper
1 teaspoon garlic powder
½ teaspoon salt
4 (6 ounce) tilapia fillets
cooking spray
2 teaspoons ground smoked paprika

Directions

1

Combine olive oil, paprika, garlic powder, salt, and black pepper in a small bowl; stir well. Brush oil mixture evenly over tilapia fillets.

2

Heat a large nonstick grill pan over medium-high heat; grease with cooking spray. Grill fish until it flakes easily with a fork, about 4 minutes per side.

Nutrition

Per Serving: 264 calories; protein 34.8g; carbohydrates 1.3g; fat 12.5g; cholesterol 61.6mg; sodium 367.2mg.

Chicken Mediterranean with Rosemary

Servings:

6

Yield:

6 servings

Ingredients

2 tablespoons white wine

3 cloves garlic, minced

½ cup diced onion

3 cups tomatoes, chopped

½ cup white wine

2 teaspoons chopped fresh thyme

2 teaspoons olive oil

6 skinless, boneless chicken breast halves

1 tablespoon chopped fresh basil

¼ cup chopped fresh parsley

salt and pepper to taste

½ cup kalamata olives

Directions

1

Heat the oil and 2 tablespoons white wine in a large skillet over medium heat. Add chicken and saute about 5 minutes each side, until golden. Remove chicken from skillet and set aside.

2

Saute garlic in pan drippings for 30 seconds, then add onion and saute for 3 minutes. Add tomatoes and bring to a boil. Lower heat, add 1/2 cup white wine and simmer for 11 minutes. Add thyme and basil and simmer for 5 more minutes.

3

Return chicken to skillet and cover. Cook over low heat until the chicken is cooked through and no longer pink inside. Add olives and parsley to the skillet and cook for 1 minute. Season with salt and pepper to taste and serve.

Nutrition

Per Serving: 222 calories; protein 28.6g; carbohydrates 7.2g; fat 6.2g; cholesterol 68.4mg; sodium 268.1mg.

Sloppy Toms

Prep:

30 mins

Cook:

1 hr 15 mins

Total:

1 hr 45 mins

Servings:

25

Yield:

5 pints

Ingredients

5 cups chopped green tomatoes

5 (1 pint) canning jars with lids and rings

2 tablespoons finely chopped crystallized ginger

1 ½ cups chopped onion

2 ¼ cups packed brown sugar

½ teaspoon salt

1 ¾ cups apple cider vinegar

1 ½ cups golden raisins

1 ½ tablespoons pickling spice

1 ½ teaspoons chili powder

1 tablespoon brown mustard seed

4 cups fresh tomatillos, husked, rinsed, and chopped

Directions

1

Place the green tomatoes, tomatillos, raisins, onion, brown sugar, salt, apple cider vinegar, pickling spice, chili powder, crystallized ginger, and brown mustard seed into a large pot over medium heat. Bring to a boil, and stir until the brown sugar has dissolved. Reduce heat, and simmer the chutney until thickened, 1 to 2 hours, stirring occasionally to keep chutney from burning on the bottom.

2

Sterilize the jars and lids in boiling water for at least 5 minutes. Pack the chutney into the hot, sterilized jars, filling the jars to within 1/4 inch of the top. Run a knife or a thin spatula around the insides of the jars after they have been filled to remove any air bubbles. Wipe the rims of the jars with a moist paper towel to remove any food residue. Top with lids, and screw on rings.

3

Place a rack in the bottom of a large stockpot and fill halfway with water. Bring to a boil over high heat, then carefully lower the jars into the pot using a holder. Leave a 2 inch space between the jars. Pour in more boiling water if necessary until the water level is at least 1 inch above the tops of the jars. Bring the water to a full boil, cover the pot, and process for 15 to 20 minutes, or the time recommended by your county Extension office.

4

Remove the jars from the stockpot and place onto a cloth-covered or wood surface, several inches apart, until cool. Once cool, press the top of each lid with a finger, ensuring that the seal is tight (lid does not move up or down at all). Store in a cool, dark area. Any uncanned chutney can be refrigerated or frozen.

Nutrition

Per Serving: 135 calories; protein 1.3g; carbohydrates 32.8g; fat 0.6g; sodium 61.2mg.

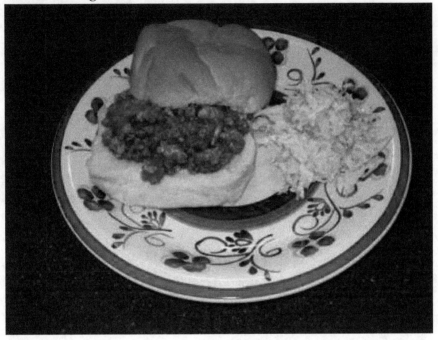

Beef Brisket

Prep:

10 mins

Cook:

4 hrs

Total:

4 hrs 10 mins

Servings:

6

Yield:

6 servings

Ingredients

1 (3 pound) beef brisket, trimmed of fat
salt and pepper to taste
1 (12 fluid ounce) can beer
1 (12 ounce) bottle tomato-based chili sauce
1 medium onion, thinly sliced
¾ cup packed brown sugar

Directions Instructions Checklist

1

Preheat the oven to 325 degrees F.

2

Season the brisket on all sides with salt and pepper, and place in a glass baking dish. Cover with a layer of sliced onions. In a medium bowl, mix together the beer, chili sauce, and brown sugar. Pour over the roast. Cover the dish tightly with aluminum foil.

3

Bake for 3 hours in the preheated oven. Remove the aluminum foil, and bake for an additional 30 minutes. Let the brisket rest and cool slightly before slicing and returning to the dish. Reheat in the oven with the sauce spooned over the sliced meat.

Nutrition

Per Serving: 520 calories; protein 23.7g; carbohydrates 32.1g; fat 31g; cholesterol 92.1mg; sodium 142.2mg.

Cinnamon Toast

Prep:

5 mins

Cook:

2 mins

Total:

7 mins

Servings:

2

Yield:

2 servings

Ingredients

2 slices white bread
2 teaspoons butter or margarine
1 teaspoon ground cinnamon
2 tablespoons white sugar

Directions

1

Use a toaster to toast the bread to desired darkness. Spread butter or margarine onto one side of each slice. In a cup or small bowl, stir together the sugar and cinnamon; sprinkle generously over hot buttered toast.

Nutrition

Per Serving: 154 calories; protein 2g; carbohydrates 26.1g; fat 4.9g; cholesterol 10.8mg; sodium 199.2mg.

Fried Rice

Prep:

10 mins

Cook:

30 mins

Additional:

20 mins

Total:

1 hr

Servings:

6

Yield:

6 servings

Ingredients

1 ½ cups uncooked jasmine rice

3 tablespoons oyster sauce

3 cups water

2 teaspoons canola oil

1 (12 ounce) can fully cooked luncheon meat (such as SPAM®), cubed

½ cup sliced Chinese sweet pork sausage (lup cheong)

3 eggs, beaten

1 (8 ounce) can pineapple chunks, drained

½ cup chopped green onion

2 tablespoons canola oil

½ teaspoon garlic powder

Directions

1

Bring the rice and water to a boil in a saucepan over high heat. Reduce heat to medium-low, cover, and simmer until the rice is tender, and the liquid has been absorbed, 20 to 25 minutes. Let the rice cool completely.

2

Heat 2 teaspoons of oil in a skillet over medium heat, and brown the luncheon meat and sausage. Set aside, and pour the beaten eggs into the hot skillet. Scramble the eggs, and set aside.

3

Heat 2 tablespoons of oil in a large nonstick skillet over medium heat, and stir in the rice. Toss the rice with the hot oil until heated through and beginning to brown, about 2 minutes. Add the garlic powder, toss the rice for 1 more minute to develop the garlic taste, and stir in the luncheon meat, sausage, scrambled eggs, pineapple, and oyster sauce. Cook and stir until the oyster sauce coats the rice and other **Ingredients**, 2 to 3 minutes, stir in the green onions, and serve.

Nutrition

Per Serving: 511 calories; protein 17.1g; carbohydrates 48g; fat 28.1g; cholesterol 132.7mg; sodium 988.1mg.

Fish Veracruz

Prep:

20 mins

Cook:

40 mins

Total:

1 hr

Servings:

8

Yield:

8 servings

Ingredients

1 tablespoon olive oil

1 onion, chopped

8 large white fish fillets

2 cloves garlic, diced

1 red bell pepper, seeded and chopped

1 cup tomato puree

1 teaspoon salt

1 cube fish bouillon

2 pounds plum tomatoes, peeled, seeded, and chopped

½ teaspoon dried oregano

¼ teaspoon ground cinnamon

2 bay leaves

20 pitted green olives

2 tablespoons capers, rinsed

freshly ground black pepper to taste

¼ cup butter

6 pickled banana peppers, sliced

Directions

1

Preheat oven to 350 degrees F. Grease a rectangular baking dish large enough to fit the fish fillets in a single layer.

2

Heat olive oil in a large saucepan over medium heat. Cook and stir onion and garlic until softened, about 5 minutes. Stir in plum tomatoes and red bell pepper; simmer until softened, about 5 minutes. Stir in tomato puree; cook for 4 minutes.

3

Stir salt, bouillon cube, oregano, cinnamon, pepper, and bay leaves into the saucepan. Cook until flavors combine, about 10-12 minutes. Add olives and capers; simmer for 5 minutes. Remove sauce from heat.

4

Melt butter in a separate skillet over medium heat. Season fish fillets with salt and pepper; cook in the hot butter until browned, 1 to 3 minutes per side.

5

Lay fish fillets in the baking dish in a single layer; cover with sauce. Arrange sliced peppers on top. Cover baking dish tightly with aluminum foil.

6

Bake in the preheated oven until fish flakes easily with a fork, 10 to 15 minutes.

Nutrition

Per Serving: 1348 calories; protein 176g; carbohydrates 11g; fat 62.5g; cholesterol 561.8mg; sodium 1606.1mg.

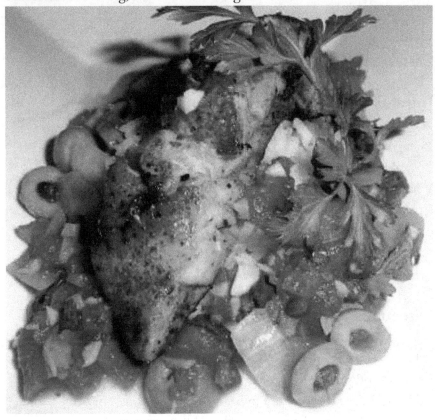

Fettuccine with Basil

Servings:

2

Yield:

2 servings

Ingredients

¾ cup chopped fresh basil

2 ½ tablespoons all-purpose flour

1 egg

1 teaspoon olive oil

2 tablespoons water

1 ½ cups all-purpose flour

Directions

1

Using a food processor, process basil leaves until chopped very fine. Add 1 1/2 cups of flour and pulse two or three times, or until combined. Add egg, 1 teaspoon oil, and the water until dough forms a ball shape. If dough seems dry, add a bit more water. Wrap dough in a piece of plastic wrap which has been coated in a few drops of olive oil. Refrigerate dough for 2 hours.

2

Remove dough from refrigerator, and cut into 6 equal size portions. Run pasta though pasta machine, or roll with rolling pin to desired thickness. Use the additional flour to coat pasta while rolling.

3

Allow pasta to dry for one hour prior to cooking.

4

Cook in a large pot of boiling water until al dente. This should take only a 3 to 6 minutes, depending on the thickness of the pasta.

Nutrition

Per Serving: 437 calories; protein 14.3g; carbohydrates 79.6g; fat 6g; cholesterol 93mg; sodium 38.2mg.

Pasta Primavera

Prep:

20 mins

Cook:

20 mins

Total:

40 mins

Servings:

4

Yield:

4 servings

Ingredients

2 cups whole grain penne pasta

½ cup freshly grated Parmesan cheese

1 tablespoon olive oil

½ cup chopped onion

2 cups sliced fresh mushrooms

1 small yellow summer squash, halved lengthwise and sliced

2 cups cherry tomatoes, halved

½ cup shredded carrot

1 pound fresh asparagus, trimmed and cut into 2-inch pieces

2 cloves garlic, minced

½ teaspoon ground black pepper

¼ teaspoon salt

⅛ teaspoon red pepper flakes

1 tablespoon chopped fresh oregano

Lemon wedges

Directions

1

Bring a large pot of lightly salted water to a boil. Add penne and cook, stirring occasionally, until tender yet firm to the bite, about 10 minutes.

2

Meanwhile, heat oil in an extra-large skillet over medium-high heat. Add onion; cook until softened, about 3 minutes. Add asparagus, mushrooms, and squash; cook until just tender, about 5 minutes. Add tomatoes, carrot, garlic, oregano, black pepper, salt, and red pepper flakes; cook until tomatoes begin to soften, about 1 minute.

3

Drain penne; stir into vegetable mixture along with 1/4 cup Parmesan cheese. Top servings with remaining cheese and serve with lemon wedges.

Nutrition

Per Serving: 281 calories; protein 15.8g; carbohydrates 41.5g; fat 7.7g; cholesterol 8.8mg; sodium 337.6mg

Polenta with Vegetables

Prep:

30 mins

Cook:

30 mins

Total:

1 hr

Servings:

6

Yield:

6 servings

Ingredients

1 (16 ounce) tube polenta, cut into 1/2 inch slices

1 (16 ounce) can black beans

1 (10 ounce) can whole kernel corn

⅓ cup black olives

1 onion, chopped

1 green bell pepper, chopped

1 (15 ounce) can kidney beans

1 small eggplant, peeled and cubed

1 (1.27 ounce) packet dry fajita seasoning

1 (8 ounce) jar salsa

1 cup shredded mozzarella cheese

6 fresh mushrooms, chopped

Directions

1

Preheat oven to 350 degrees F. Lightly oil a 9x13 inch baking dish.

2

Heat oil in a skillet over medium heat. Cook and stir onion, green pepper, eggplant, and mushrooms in oil until soft. Mix in fajita seasoning.

3

Line prepared baking dish with slices of polenta. Spread beans and corn evenly over the polenta, and then spread onion mixture over the beans. Top with salsa, mozzarella cheese and black olives.

4

Bake until heated through, about 20 minutes.

Nutrition

Per Serving: 329 calories; protein 17.8g; carbohydrates 57.5g; fat 5g; cholesterol 12.1mg; sodium 1633.4mg.

Pasta with Pumpkin Sauce

Prep:

10 mins

Cook:

30 mins

Total:

40 mins

Servings:

4

Yield:

4 servings

Ingredients

¼ cup butter, divided

salt and freshly ground black pepper to taste

1 pound sugar pumpkin - peeled, seeded, and cut into small cubes

½ pound orecchiette pasta

1 cup heavy cream

4 tablespoons Parmesan cheese

2 orange bell peppers, seeded and diced

1 onion, minced

Directions

1

Melt 1/2 the butter in a large skillet over medium-low heat and cook onion until soft and translucent, about 5 minutes. Add pumpkin and cook for 2 minutes. Cover, reduce heat, and cook, stirring often, until soft, about 28-30 minutes.

2

Meanwhile, bring a large pot of lightly salted water to a boil. Cook orecchiette in the boiling water, stirring occasionally until almost tender yet firm to the bite, about 10 minutes, 2 minutes less than indicated on the package. Drain and transfer to a bowl.

3

Melt the remaining butter in a second skillet and cook bell peppers until softened, 5 to 10 minutes. Add to the bowl with the cooked pasta.

4

Once pumpkin is tender, add cream and Parmesan cheese to skillet. Season with salt and pepper and stir until smooth. Add drained pasta and cooked bell peppers and mix well.

Nutrition

Per Serving: 581 calories; protein 12g; carbohydrates 55.5g; fat 36.1g; cholesterol 116.4mg; sodium 222.9mg.

Mexican Bake

Servings:

6

Yield:

6 servings

Ingredients

1 ½ cups cooked rice, preferably brown

1 cup chopped poblano pepper

2 (14.5 ounce) cans no-salt-added tomatoes, diced or crushed

1 (15 ounce) can no-salt-added black beans, drained and rinsed

1 cup frozen yellow corn kernels

1 cup chopped red bell pepper

1 cup shredded reduced-fat Monterey Jack cheese

1 tablespoon chili powder

1 tablespoon cumin

4 garlic cloves, crushed

1 pound skinless, boneless chicken breast, cut in bite-sized pieces

Directions

1

Preheat oven to 400 degrees. Spread rice in a shallow 3-quart casserole. Top with chicken. In a bowl, combine tomatoes, beans, corn, peppers, seasonings and garlic; pour over chicken. Top with cheese and optional jalapeno. Bake 45 minutes.

Nutrition

Per Serving: 325 calories; protein 28.4g; carbohydrates 36.9g; fat 7.1g; cholesterol 56.5mg; sodium 355.8mg.

Pasta Soup

Prep:

15 mins

Cook:

25 mins

Total:

40 mins

Servings:

4

Yield:

4 servings

Ingredients

¾ pound Italian sausage

2 tablespoons chopped fresh basil

½ cup diced onion

6 cups chicken broth

¼ teaspoon ground black pepper

5 ounces farfalle pasta

½ teaspoon Italian seasoning

½ teaspoon salt, or to taste

½ cup ricotta cheese

½ cup shredded mozzarella cheese

¼ cup freshly grated Parmesan cheese

1 (15 ounce) can diced tomatoes with basil, garlic, and oregano

Directions

1

Cook Italian sausage and onion in a skillet over medium-high heat until sausage is browned and crumbly and onion is soft and translucent, about 7 minutes.

2

Mix in chicken broth, diced tomatoes, pasta, Italian seasoning, salt, and pepper. Bring to a boil. Reduce heat and simmer until pasta is tender, stirring occasionally, about 10 minutes. Add ricotta cheese and cook until ricotta is fully incorporated, 2 to 3 minutes more.

3

Top each serving with 2 tablespoons mozzarella cheese, 1 tablespoon Parmesan cheese, and 1/2 tablespoon fresh basil.

Nutrition

Per Serving: 482 calories; protein 27.4g; carbohydrates 37.5g; fat 23.7g; cholesterol 64.7mg; sodium 3111.4mg.

Cranberry Relish

Prep:

20 mins

Additional:

1 day

Total:

1 day

Servings:

40

Yield:

2 1/2 pints

Ingredients

1 ½ pounds fresh cranberries

¼ cup cranberry juice

2 pears - peeled, cored, and quartered

2 oranges - zested, peeled, and segmented

2 lemons - zested, peeled, and segmented

2 Granny Smith apples - peeled, cored, and quartered

¾ cup white sugar

¼ cup brandy

Directions

1

Combine cranberries, pears, apples, oranges, and lemons in a food processor; grind to a fine consistency. Transfer to a large glass bowl. Stir sugar, orange zest, and lemon zest into the fruit mixture. Add brandy and cranberry juice; stir.

2

Cover bowl with plastic wrap and refrigerate for at least 24 hours.

Nutrition

Per Serving: 35 calories; protein 0.1g; carbohydrates 8.2g; sodium 0.5mg.

Grilled Cod

Prep:

10 mins

Cook:

10 mins

Additional:

15 mins

Total:

35 mins

Servings:

4

Yield:

4 servings

Ingredients

2 (8 ounce) fillets cod, cut in half

¼ teaspoon ground black pepper

1 tablespoon Cajun seasoning

½ teaspoon lemon pepper

¼ teaspoon salt

2 tablespoons chopped green onion (white part only)

2 tablespoons butter

1 lemon, juiced

Directions

1

Stack about 15 charcoal briquettes into a grill in a pyramid shape. If desired, drizzle coals lightly with lighter fluid and allow to soak for 1 minute before lighting coals with a match. Allow fire to spread to all coals, about 10 minutes, before spreading briquettes out into the grill; let coals burn until a thin layer of white ash covers the coals. Lightly oil the grates.

2

Season both sides of cod with Cajun seasoning, lemon pepper, salt, and black pepper. Set fish aside on a plate. Heat butter in a small saucepan over medium heat, stir in lemon juice and green onion, and cook until onion is softened, about 3-5 minutes.

3

Place cod onto oiled grates and grill until fish is browned and flakes easily, about 3 minutes per side; baste with butter mixture frequently while grilling. Allow cod to rest off the heat for about 5 minutes before serving.

Nutrition

Per Serving: 152 calories; protein 20.3g; carbohydrates 2.2g; fat 6.6g; cholesterol 63.4mg; sodium 660.6mg.

Herbed Sole

Prep:

15 mins

Cook:

30 mins

Total:

45 mins

Servings:

4

Yield:

4 servings

Ingredients

1 tablespoon lemon juice

1 tablespoon all-purpose flour

2 tablespoons thinly sliced green onion

1 clove garlic, minced

¼ cup dry white wine

4 (6 ounce) fillets sole

salt to taste

ground black pepper to taste

¼ teaspoon paprika

¼ pound cooked salad shrimp

2 tablespoons butter

Directions

1

In a small bowl, combine lemon juice, green onion, garlic, and wine. Set aside.

2

Lay filets flat, and divide shrimp evenly among them in a band across one end of each fillet. Roll up around shrimp, and secure with toothpick. Place in a baking dish. Season to taste with salt, pepper, and paprika. Pour lemon juice mixture over the fish. Cover.

3

Bake at 350 degrees F for 25 minutes.

4

When fillets are nearly done, prepare sauce. In a small saucepan, melt butter over medium heat. Stir in flour. Transfer fish to serving platter ,and keep warm. Pour pan juices into butter/flour mixture; cook and stir until thickened. Pour over sole, and serve.

Nutrition

Per Serving: 253 calories; protein 37.5g; carbohydrates 2.8g; fat 8.1g; cholesterol 149.9mg; sodium 226.5mg.

Grilled Salmon with Bacon and Corn Relish

Prep:

20 mins

Cook:

25 mins

Total:

45 mins

Servings:

2

Yield:

2 servings

Ingredients

6 slices bacon, cut crosswise into 1/2-inch pieces

2 ears white corn

1 pinch cayenne pepper

¼ cup chopped green onions - white and light green parts separated from green tops

¼ cup diced red bell pepper

salt and ground black pepper to taste

2 teaspoons olive oil

1 tablespoon rice vinegar

½ teaspoon vegetable oil

2 (8 ounce) center-cut boneless salmon fillets

1 pinch cayenne pepper

Directions

1

Preheat an outdoor grill (for high heat and lightly oil the grate.

2

Place bacon in a skillet over medium heat and cook until browned and crisp, 8 to 10 minutes.

3

Cut kernels from corn ears into a large bowl using a sharp knife held at a 45-degree angle. Scrape cobs with the back of the knife into the bowl to get the juices.

4

Stir white and light green parts of green onions into bacon and add red bell pepper; cook and stir until vegetables just start to become tender, about 2 minutes. Stir corn into bacon mixture and let corn just warm through. Season with salt, black pepper, cayenne pepper, a few chopped dark green onion tops, olive oil, and rice vinegar. Turn off heat under relish.

5

Spread vegetable oil onto both sides of salmon fillets and season fish with salt, black pepper, and cayenne pepper.

6

Cook on preheated grill until fish shows good grill marks, the flesh flakes easily, and fish is still slightly pink in the center, about 5 minutes per side. A crack that opens up in the salmon flesh as you cook will let you see how done the salmon is in the middle.

7

Divide spinach leaves onto 2 plates and top each with a salmon fillet and half the bacon relish. Sprinkle on a few green onion tops for garnish.

Nutrition

Per Serving: 605 calories; protein 56.6g; carbohydrates 20.2g; fat 33.1g; cholesterol 140.8mg; sodium 754.8mg.

Sirloin Marinara

Prep:

15 mins

Cook:

15 mins

Total:

30 mins

Servings:

8

Yield:

8 servings

Ingredients

2 tablespoons olive oil

2 pounds top sirloin steak, sliced

2 cups chunky pasta sauce

1 onion, thinly sliced

½ cup red wine

2 cloves garlic, minced

Directions

1

Heat the oil in a 10 inch skillet over medium high heat. Add the onions and saute until tender, about 5 minutes. Add the steak strips, turning so that all sides get browned, about 10 minutes.

2

Add the tomato sauce, garlic and red wine. Reduce heat to low and simmer for 11 to 15 minutes, or until the steak is cooked through.

Nutrition

Per Serving: 276 calories; protein 20g; carbohydrates 10.5g; fat 15.4g; cholesterol 61.7mg; sodium 299.9mg.

Taco Chicken Salad

Prep:

20 mins

Cook:

30 mins

Total:

50 mins

Servings:

4

Yield:

4 servings

Ingredients

1 ½ tablespoons paprika

1 ½ teaspoons cayenne pepper

1 ½ teaspoons garlic powder

1 teaspoon ground black pepper

1 teaspoon ground white pepper

¾ teaspoon ground cumin

1 ½ teaspoons onion powder

¾ teaspoon dried oregano

¾ teaspoon dried thyme

4 skinless, boneless chicken breast halves

1 tablespoon vegetable oil

4 tostada shells

¾ teaspoon salt

2 cups chopped romaine lettuce

2 cups fresh salsa

½ cup sliced black olives

½ cup ranch dressing

2 avocados - peeled, pitted, and sliced
½ cup shredded Cheddar cheese

Directions

1

Preheat oven to 350 degrees F.

2

Stir paprika, cayenne pepper, garlic powder, onion powder, black pepper, white pepper, cumin, oregano, thyme, and salt together in a bowl.

3

Rub spice mixture into each chicken breast to coat thoroughly.

4

Heat oil in a large skillet over high heat. Cook chicken breasts in hot oil until browned, about 5 minutes per side. Transfer chicken to a baking dish. Cover the dish with aluminum foil.

5

Bake in the preheated oven until chicken breasts are no longer pink in the center and the juices run clear, about 20 minutes. An instant-read thermometer inserted into the center should read at least 165 degrees F. Slice chicken into strips.

6

Fill each tostada shell with 1/2 cup lettuce. Divide chicken, salsa, avocados, Cheddar cheese, and olives between the tostada shells. Top each salad with ranch dressing.

Nutrition

Per Serving: 667 calories; protein 33.9g; carbohydrates 33.2g; fat 47g; cholesterol 87.6mg; sodium 1861.3mg.

Cucumber Salad

Prep:

15 mins

Additional:

20 mins

Total:

35 mins

Servings:

8

Yield:

8 servings

Ingredients

2 large cucumbers, peeled and sliced

2 tablespoons white vinegar

1 ½ tablespoons sour cream

1 teaspoon salt

½ cup diced sweet onion (such as Vidalia®)

½ teaspoon cracked black pepper

2 tablespoons white sugar

Directions

1

Combine cucumbers, onion, vinegar, sugar, sour cream, salt, and pepper together in a bowl.

2

Cover bowl with plastic wrap and refrigerate until chilled, 20 to 30 minutes.

Nutrition

Per Serving: 31 calories; protein 0.6g; carbohydrates 6.1g; fat 0.7g;
cholesterol 1.2mg; sodium 294mg.

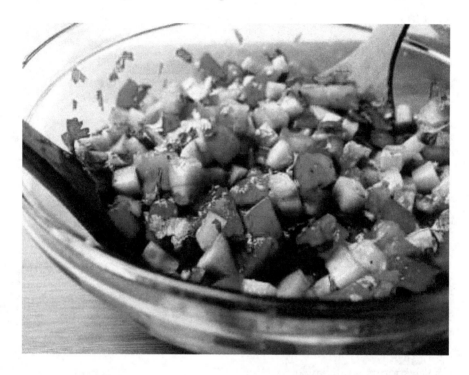

Egg Cheese Quiche

Prep:

30 mins

Cook:

1 hr

Total:

1 hr 30 mins

Servings:

6

Yield:

1 (9 inch) quiche

Ingredients

1 tablespoon butter

1 (12 ounce) package spicy ground pork sausage

4 eggs

1 (8 ounce) package Cheddar cheese, shredded

½ cup Ranch-style salad dressing

½ cup milk

1 dash hot pepper sauce

salt and pepper to taste

1 pinch white sugar

1 (9 inch) unbaked deep dish pie crust

½ onion, chopped

Directions

1

Preheat oven to 425 degrees F.

2

Heat butter in a large skillet over medium heat. Saute onion until soft. Add sausage, and cook until evenly brown. Drain, crumble, and set aside.

3

In a medium bowl, whisk together eggs, Ranch dressing and milk. Stir in shredded cheese. Season with hot sauce, salt, pepper and sugar.

4

Spread sausage mixture in the bottom of crust. Cover with egg mixture, and shake lightly to remove air, and to level contents.

5

Bake in preheated oven for 15 to 20 minutes. Reduce heat to 350 degrees F, and bake 45 to 50 minutes, or until filling is puffed and golden brown. Remove from oven, prick top with a knife, and let cool 10 minutes before serving.

Nutrition

Per Serving: 718 calories; protein 22.5g; carbohydrates 19.3g; fat 60.9g; cholesterol 213.4mg; sodium 1450.6mg.

Cereal with Fruit

Prep:

10 mins

Cook:

45 mins

Additional:

5 mins

Total:

1 hr

Servings:

16

Yield:

4 cups

Ingredients

¾ cup brown sugar

¼ cup water

2 teaspoons ground cinnamon

½ teaspoon salt

1 cup chopped walnuts

1 tablespoon honey

2 teaspoons vanilla extract

3 cups rolled oats

Directions

1

Preheat an oven to 275 degrees F. Cover a 10x15 inch pan with wax paper.

2

Mix brown sugar and water in a microwave safe bowl. Cook in microwave to dissolve the sugar, about 1 minute. Combine oats, salt, walnuts, and cinnamon in a large bowl. Stir in sugar mixture, honey, and vanilla extract. Mix well. Pour mixture onto the prepared pan, spreading evenly. Create clusters by squeezing small handfuls of the oat mixture together.

3

Bake in the preheated oven for 20 minutes. Remove from oven and gently stir granola using a spoon. Return to the oven and bake for an additional 25 minutes. The granola will be slightly browned and will continue to harden as they cool.

Nutrition

Per Serving: 139 calories; protein 3.2g; carbohydrates 19.4g; fat 5.9g; sodium 75.9mg.

Beef Tacos

Prep:

15 mins

Additional:

30 mins

Total:

45 mins

Servings:

6

Yield:

6 servings

Ingredients

PAM® Original No-Stick Cooking Spray

1 pound ground chuck beef (80% lean)

2 cups frozen Southwest mixed vegetables (corn, black beans, red peppers)

1 (10 ounce) can Ro*Tel® Original Diced Tomatoes & Green Chilies, undrained

1 (10 ounce) can red enchilada sauce

6 ounces dry extra-wide egg noodles, uncooked

1 ¼ cups water

¼ cup thinly sliced green onions

1 teaspoon Sour cream

1 ¼ cups shredded Mexican blend cheese

Directions

1

Preheat oven to 400 degrees F.

2

Spray 13x9-inch glass baking dish with cooking spray. Place uncooked noodles in baking dish.

3

Heat large skillet over medium-high heat. Add beef; cook 6-7 minutes or until crumbled and no longer pink. Drain. Add vegetables, undrained tomatoes, enchilada sauce and water to skillet; stir. Bring to a boil. Pour mixture over noodles.

4

Cover dish tightly with foil; bake 15 minutes. Stir; sprinkle with cheese and cover with foil. Bake 10 minutes more or until noodles are tender. Sprinkle with green onions. Serve with sour cream, if desired.

Nutrition

Per Serving: 474 calories; protein 25.8g; carbohydrates 30.9g; fat 27g; cholesterol 107.6mg; sodium 656.6mg.

CHAPTER 4: SNACK & APPETIZER

Pita Pizza

Prep:

5 mins

Cook:

15 mins

Total:

20 mins

Servings:

1

Yield:

1 serving

Ingredients

1 teaspoon olive oil
3 tablespoons pizza sauce
¼ cup sliced crimini mushrooms
⅛ teaspoon garlic salt
½ cup shredded mozzarella cheese
1 pita bread round

Directions

1

Preheat grill for medium-high heat.

2

Spread one side of the pita with olive oil and pizza sauce. Top with cheese and mushrooms, and season with garlic salt.

3

Lightly oil grill grate. Place pita pizza on grill, cover, and cook until cheese completely melts, about 5 minutes.

Nutrition

Per Serving: 405 calories; protein 19.7g; carbohydrates 39.9g; fat 18g; cholesterol 44.2mg; sodium 1155.9mg.

Avocado Dip

Prep:

30 mins

Cook:

13 mins

Total:

43 mins

Servings:

3

Yield:

3 servings

Ingredients

2 Hass avocado, peeled and pitted
2 green plantains, peeled and sliced into fifths
1 tablespoon lemon juice
¼ teaspoon salt
1 clove garlic, minced
vegetable oil for frying
1 tablespoon mayonnaise

Directions

1

Combine avocados, lemon juice, mayonnaise, and salt together in a bowl; sprinkle in garlic. Mash using a potato masher until dip is creamy.

2

Heat oil in a deep-fryer or large saucepan to 350 degrees F. Drizzle about 1 teaspoon oil onto a clean work surface and the bottom of a coffee cup.

3

Fry the plantains in the hot oil until golden brown, 8 to 10 minutes. Remove from fryer and place on the work surface; flatten with the bottom of the coffee cup. Re-fry until browned and tender, about 5 minutes. Place on a paper towel-covered plate; sprinkle with salt. Serve plantains alongside the dip.

Nutrition

Per Serving: 830 calories; protein 1.7g; carbohydrates 39g; fat 77.4g; cholesterol 1.7mg; sodium 224.9mg.

Artichoke Dip

Prep:

5 mins

Cook:

20 mins

Total:

25 mins

Servings:

7

Yield:

5 to 8 servings

Ingredients

½ cup mayonnaise

½ cup sour cream

salt and pepper to taste

1 (14 ounce) can artichoke hearts, drained

½ cup minced red onion

1 cup grated Parmesan cheese

1 tablespoon lemon juice

Directions

1

Preheat oven to 400 degrees F.

2

In a medium-sized mixing bowl, stir together mayonnaise, sour cream, Parmesan cheese and onion. When these ingredients are combined, mix in artichoke hearts, lemon juice, salt and pepper. Transfer mixture to a shallow baking dish.

3

Bake at 400 degrees F for 20 minutes, or until light brown on top.

Nutrition

Per Serving: 221 calories; protein 6.4g; carbohydrates 6.6g; fat 19.2g; cholesterol 23.3mg; sodium 481.4mg.

Hummus

Prep:

10 mins

Total:

10 mins

Servings:

8

Yield:

8 servings

Ingredients

2 (15 ounce) cans garbanzo beans, drained and liquid reserved

5 tablespoons lemon juice

3 cloves garlic

1 teaspoon salt

1 teaspoon ground coriander

⅛ teaspoon cayenne pepper

6 tablespoons olive oil

⅛ teaspoon ground cumin

Directions

1

Combine garbanzo beans, olive oil, lemon juice, garlic, salt, coriander, cumin, and cayenne in a food processor. Add 4 tablespoons reserved bean liquid and process until hummus is smooth.

Nutrition

Per Serving: 177 calories; protein 3.6g; carbohydrates 16.6g; fat 11g; sodium 500.5mg.

Shrimp Ceviche

Prep:

15 mins

Cook:

5 mins

Additional:

20 mins

Total:

40 mins

Servings:

4

Yield:

4 servings

Ingredients

1 cucumber, diced
½ pound raw shrimp, peeled and deveined
2 Roma tomatoes, diced
1 ½ teaspoons salt, divided
½ medium red onion, diced
2 serrano peppers, seeded and deveined
¼ cup chopped cilantro
6 medium limes, divided
½ teaspoon ground black pepper to taste

Directions

1

Combine cucumber, tomatoes, red onion, serrano peppers, and cilantro in a bowl. Add 1 teaspoon salt and squeeze 1 lime. Gently mix and set aside.

2

Squeeze the remaining limes into another bowl. Add remaining salt and pepper.

3

Bring a 1- to 2-quart pot of water to a boil. Place shrimp into the boiling water for 45 seconds. Quickly remove from the water using a strainer.

4

Chop the partially cooked shrimp into small pieces and add to the bowl with the seasoned lime mixture. Let sit for 20 minutes. Combine with the cucumber mixture and top with avocados.

Nutrition

Per Serving: 163 calories; protein 11.7g; carbohydrates 19g; fat 7.1g; cholesterol 86.3mg; sodium 981mg.

Pickled Asparagus

Prep:

10 mins

Cook:

5 mins

Total:

15 mins

Servings:

10

Yield:

1 quart

Ingredients

1 bunch fresh asparagus spears
2 tablespoons Old Bay Seasoning TM
2 bay leaves
1 cup water
1 cup white wine vinegar
¼ cup brown sugar
4 cloves garlic, crushed
6 whole black peppercorns
1 jalapeno pepper, seeded and julienned
4 sprigs fresh thyme
1 teaspoon salt

Directions

1

Trim the bottoms off of the asparagus, and pack loosely into a 1 quart jar.

2

Combine the water, white wine vinegar, brown sugar, garlic, jalapeno, thyme sprigs, bay leaves, salt and whole peppercorns in a saucepan. Bring to a boil, and boil hard for 1 minute.

3

Pour the hot liquid over the asparagus in the jar, filling to cover the tips of the asparagus. Cover, and cool to room temperature. Store in the refrigerator for 24 hours to blend flavors before serving.

Nutrition

Per Serving: 37 calories; protein 1.3g; carbohydrates 8.5g; fat 0.2g; sodium 564.9mg.

Baba Ghanoush

Prep:

5 mins

Cook:

40 mins

Additional:

3 hrs

Total:

3 hrs 45 mins

Servings:

12

Yield:

1 1/2 cups

Ingredients

1 eggplant
¼ cup lemon juice
2 cloves garlic, minced
salt and pepper to taste
1 ½ tablespoons olive oil
¼ cup tahini
2 tablespoons sesame seeds

Directions

1

Preheat oven to 400 degrees F. Lightly grease a baking sheet.

2

Place eggplant on baking sheet, and make holes in the skin with a fork. Roast it for 30 to 40 minutes, turning occasionally, or until soft. Remove from oven, and place into a large bowl of cold water. Remove from water, and peel skin off.

3

Place eggplant, lemon juice, tahini, sesame seeds, and garlic in an electric blender, and puree. Season with salt and pepper to taste. Transfer eggplant mixture to a medium size mixing bowl, and slowly mix in olive oil. Refrigerate for 3 hours before serving.

Nutrition

Per Serving: 66 calories; protein 1.6g; carbohydrates 4.6g; fat 5.2g; sodium 7mg.

Walnuts Pesto

Prep:

10 mins

Total:

10 mins

Servings:

2

Yield:

2 servings

Ingredients

½ cup walnuts

2 cloves garlic

1 tablespoon lemon juice

¼ cup olive oil

2 cups basil leaves

Directions

1

Blend basil, walnuts, olive oil, garlic, and lemon juice together in a food processor until pesto has a paste-like consistency.

Nutrition

Per Serving: 455 calories; protein 6.1g; carbohydrates 6.9g; fat 47.3g; sodium 2.9mg.

Vegetable Dill Dip

Prep:

10 mins

Additional:

4 hrs

Total:

4 hrs 10 mins

Servings:

16

Yield:

2 cups

Ingredients

1 cup sour cream

1 cup mayonnaise

1 teaspoon Beau Monde ™ seasoning

1 tablespoon dried dill weed

1 tablespoon minced onion

1 tablespoon dried parsley

Directions

1

Stir the sour cream, mayonnaise, dill, onion, parsley, and Beau Monde ™ seasoning in a bowl. Cover and refrigerate 4 hours or overnight.

Nutrition

Per Serving: 131 calories; protein 0.6g; carbohydrates 1.3g; fat 13.9g; cholesterol 11.5mg; sodium 116.9mg.

Acai Bowl

Prep:

10 mins

Total:

10 mins

Servings:

1

Yield:

1 bowl

Ingredients

1 cup acai berry sorbet

2 tablespoons granola

1 banana

2 teaspoons unsweetened coconut flakes

1 teaspoon honey

4 strawberries, sliced

Directions

1

Place acai sorbet in a bowl and top with a layer of granola. Line strawberries and bananas on granola layer and top with coconut and a drizzle of honey.

Nutrition

Per Serving: 551 calories; protein 4.3g; carbohydrates 107.7g; fat 12.8g; sodium 27.5mg.

Almond Bars

Prep:

10 mins

Cook:

10 mins

Additional:

5 mins

Total:

25 mins

Servings:

48

Yield:

48 bars

Ingredients

12 graham crackers
1 teaspoon vanilla extract
¾ cup butter
1 cup brown sugar
1 cup sliced almonds

Directions

1

Preheat oven to 350 degrees F. Grease a 10x15 inch jelly roll pan.

2

Break graham crackers into 4 pieces and arrange them touching on the prepared jelly roll pan. Sprinkle the sliced almonds over the crackers.

In a small saucepan, melt butter. When butter is melted, stir in the brown sugar and vanilla until smooth and remove from heat. Pour the butter mixture evenly over the graham crackers in the pan.

3

Bake for 8 to 10 minutes in the preheated oven. Watch carefully so that the edges do not burn. Cut bars while still warm and remove from pan. If the bars are stuck, put the pan into the warm oven for a minute to loosen.

Nutrition

Per Serving: 63 calories; protein 0.7g; carbohydrates 6.1g; fat 4.2g; cholesterol 7.6mg; sodium 42.5mg.

CHAPTER 5: SMOOTHIES & DRINK RECIPES

Berries Smoothie

Prep:

5 mins

Total:

5 mins

Servings:

2

Yield:

2 servings

Ingredients

1 cup Almond Breeze Vanilla or Unsweetened Vanilla almondmilk

½ cup fresh raspberries

½ cup fresh blueberries

½ cup fresh blackberries

Directions

1

Puree all Ingredients in a blender until smooth.

Nutrition:

Calories 100

Total Fat 1.5

Cholesterol 0mg

Sodium 75

Cherry Smoothie

Prep:

5 mins

Total:

5 mins

Servings:

1

Yield:

1 smoothie

Ingredients

1 cup frozen strawberries

½ cup frozen dark sweet cherries

½ cup nonfat plain yogurt

½ cup ice cubes

½ cup cold almond milk

Directions

1

Combine strawberries, yogurt, almond milk, and frozen cherries in a blender; add ice. Blend until smooth, about 1 minute.

Nutrition

Per Serving: 275 calories; protein 8g; carbohydrates 62.9g; fat 1.7g; cholesterol 2.5mg; sodium 153.1mg.

Pineapple Juice

Prep:

5 mins

Total:

5 mins

Servings:

14

Yield:

14 (8 ounce) servings

Ingredients

1 (64 fluid ounce) bottle cranberry juice, chilled

1 (8 ounce) can pineapple tidbits

1 cup cranberries

1 (46 fluid ounce) can pineapple juice

Directions

1

In a punch bowl, combine cranberry juice and pineapple juice. Stir in pineapple tidbits and cranberries. Serve with ice.

Nutrition

Per Serving: 134 calories; protein 0.4g; carbohydrates 33.2g; fat 0.3g; sodium 4.8mg.

Healthy Coffee Smoothie

Prep:

5 mins

Total:

5 mins

Servings:

1

Yield:

1 smoothie

Ingredients

1 cup brewed coffee

2 tablespoons coconut oil, melted

2 large pasteurized egg yolks

1 tablespoon coconut sugar

¼ cup avocado

¼ cup ice cubes

Directions

1

Combine coffee, egg yolks, avocado, ice cubes, and coconut sugar in a blender; blend until smooth. Add coconut oil and blend until smooth.

Nutrition

Per Serving: 486 calories; protein 6.7g; carbohydrates 19.4g; fat 44.5g; cholesterol 409.7mg; sodium 30.4mg.

Green Delight

Prep:

5 mins

Total:

5 mins

Servings:

1

Yield:

1 glass

Ingredients

½ cup frozen blueberries

2 cups iced green tea

4 frozen strawberries

Directions

1

Place the blueberries and strawberries in the bottom of a tall glass. Pour the green tea over the berries.

Nutrition

Per Serving: 59 calories; protein 0.5g; carbohydrates 14.7g; fat 0.6g; sodium 15.8mg.

Vanille Kipferl

Prep:

30 mins

Cook:

8 mins

Additional:

2 mins

Total:

40 mins

Servings:

18

Yield:

3 dozen

Ingredients

2 cups all-purpose flour

¼ cup confectioners' sugar

⅓ cup white sugar

1 cup unsalted butter

¼ cup vanilla sugar

¾ cup ground almonds

Directions

1

Preheat oven to 325 degrees F. Line a baking sheet with parchment paper.

2

Combine flour, 1/3 cup sugar, and ground almonds. Cut in butter with pastry blender, then quickly knead into a dough.

3

Shape dough into logs and cut off 1/2-inch pieces. Shape each piece into a crescent and place on prepared baking sheet.

4

Bake in preheated oven until edges are golden brown, 8 to 10 minutes. Cool 1 minute and carefully roll in vanilla sugar mixture.

Nutrition

Per Serving: 207 calories; protein 2.8g; carbohydrates 20g; fat 13.4g; cholesterol 27.1mg; sodium 1.8mg.

Banana Supreme Shake

Prep:

5 mins

Total:

5 mins

Servings:

1

Yield:

1 serving

Ingredients

1 (8 ounce) container Classic French Vanilla Flavor Ready-to-Drink
CARNATION BREAKFAST ESSENTIALS® Complete Nutritional
Drink
1 banana
4 ice cubes
1 tablespoon instant coffee crystals

Directions

1

Place all ingredients in blender; cover. Blend until smooth. Pour into
glass and enjoy!

Nutrition

Per Serving: 351 calories; protein 11.6g; carbohydrates 69g; fat 4.4g;
cholesterol 10mg; sodium 154.6mg.

Melon Chiller

Prep:

20 mins

Total:

20 mins

Servings:

10

Yield:

10 servings

Ingredients

1 cantaloupe, halved and seeded
2 cups white sugar
ice cubes, as needed
1 gallon water

Directions

1

Scrape the cantaloupe meat lengthwise with a spoon or a melon baller
and place in a punch bowl; add the water and sugar. Mix thoroughly
until all the sugar is dissolved. Chill with the addition of plenty of ice
cubes.

Nutrition

Per Serving: 174 calories; protein 0.5g; carbohydrates 44.5g; fat 0.1g;
sodium 20.2mg.

Banana and Almond Muffin

Prep:

10 mins

Cook:

20 mins

Total:

30 mins

Servings:

20

Yield:

20 muffins

Ingredients

6 large ripe bananas
2 teaspoons baking powder
1 cup brown sugar
¾ cup salted butter, melted
2 eggs
1 ½ cups all-purpose flour
1 ¼ cups whole wheat flour
½ cup ground flax seeds
½ cup white sugar
2 teaspoons baking soda

Directions

1

Preheat oven to 350 degrees F. Line 2 muffin tins with paper liners.

2

Mash bananas in a bowl. Add brown sugar, butter, white sugar, and eggs; mix well. Add all-purpose flour, whole wheat flour, flax seeds, baking soda, and baking powder. Scoop batter into the prepared tins.

3

Bake in the preheated oven until tops spring back when lightly pressed, about 20 minutes.

Nutrition

Per Serving: 240 calories; protein 3.7g; carbohydrates 38.7g; fat 8.9g; cholesterol 36.9mg; sodium 235.5mg.

Coconut Smoothie

Prep:

10 mins

Total:

10 mins

Servings:

2

Yield:

2 smoothies

Ingredients

2 bananas

1 cup water

⅓ cup coconut milk

1 tablespoon almond butter

1 tablespoon moringa powder

1 cup sliced frozen peaches

Directions

1

Layer bananas, peaches, coconut milk, moringa powder, and almond butter in a blender; add water. Blend mixture until very smooth, at least 1 minute.

Nutrition

Per Serving: 252 calories; protein 4g; carbohydrates 34.7g; fat 13.2g; sodium 48.2mg

Mango & Lime Smoothie

Prep:

10 mins

Total:

10 mins

Servings:

4

Yield:

4 servings

Ingredients

2 tablespoons confectioners' sugar

1 tray ice cubes

2 tablespoons fresh lime juice

3 mangoes, peeled, pitted, and cut into 1-inch chunks

Directions

1

Place the mangoes, lime juice, confectioners' sugar, and ice cubes in a blender. Blend until slushy.

Nutrition

Per Serving: 117 calories; protein 0.8g; carbohydrates 30.7g; fat 0.4g; sodium 5.8mg.

CHAPTER 6: DESSERTS

Frozen Mango Bellini

Prep:

5 mins

Total:

5 mins

Servings:

1

Yield:

1 cocktail

Ingredients

1 ½ fluid ounces mango juice
1 sprig fresh mint
½ fluid ounce orange-flavored liqueur (such as Cointreau®)
10 ounces ice cubes
3 fluid ounces Prosecco (such as Caposaldo DOC)

Directions

1

Pour mango juice, Prosecco, and orange liqueur into a blender in the order listed; add ice. Blend until smooth. Pour into a serving glass. Garnish with mint.

Nutrition

Per Serving: 208 calories; protein 0.3g; carbohydrates 22.2g; fat 0.1g; sodium 19.7mg.

Cherry Frozen Yogurt

Prep:

25 mins

Additional:

4 hrs

Total:

4 hrs 25 mins

Servings:

12

Yield:

6 cups

Ingredients

1 (8 ounce) package cream cheese, softened

1 cup white sugar

1 tablespoon lemon juice

2 cups pitted, chopped fresh cherries

3 cups plain Greek yogurt

Directions

1

In a large bowl, mash the cream cheese with sugar until thoroughly combined; stir in the lemon juice, and mix in the yogurt, about a cup at a time, until the mixture is smooth and creamy. Mix in the cherries. Cover the bowl with plastic wrap, and chill until very cold, at least 4 hours.

2

Pour the mixture into an ice cream freezer, and freeze according to manufacturer's instructions. For firmer texture, pack the frozen yogurt into a covered container, and freeze for several hours.

Nutrition

Per Serving: 212 calories; protein 4.7g; carbohydrates 23.3g; fat 11.7g; cholesterol 31.8mg; sodium 87.8mg

Ricotta Mousse

Prep:

10 mins

Cook:

5 mins

Total:

15 mins

Servings:

6

Yield:

6 servings

Ingredients

3 ounces unsweetened chocolate, cut into small pieces

1 teaspoon vanilla extract

⅓ cup honey

1 pound ricotta cheese

Directions

1

Place chocolate in the top of a double boiler over simmering water. Stir frequently, scraping down the sides with a rubber spatula to avoid scorching, until chocolate is melted, about 5 minutes. Allow to cool slightly.

2

Combine melted chocolate, ricotta cheese, honey, and vanilla extract in a blender; blend until smooth. Pour into dessert cups or glasses and let chill completely.

Nutrition

Per Serving: 230 calories; protein 9.4g; carbohydrates 29g; fat 9.7g; cholesterol 23.5mg; sodium 99.1mg.

Avocado Pudding

Prep:

5 mins

Additional:

1 hr

Total:

1 hr 5 mins

Servings:

1

Yield:

1 serving

Ingredients

1 ripe avocado
2 packets stevia sugar substitute (such as Truvia®)
⅓ cup heavy cream
1 pinch salt
½ teaspoon vanilla extract

Directions

1

Combine avocado, cream, sweetener, vanilla extract, and salt in a
blender; blend until smooth. Chill for 1 hour.

Nutrition

Per Serving: 604 calories; protein 5.6g; carbohydrates 21.6g; fat 58.8g;
cholesterol 108.7mg; sodium 199.4mg.

Apple Crisp

Prep:

20 mins

Cook:

35 mins

Additional:

45 mins

Total:

1 hr 40 mins

Servings:

4

Yield:

4 servings

Ingredients

4 apples - peeled, cored, and sliced
1 teaspoon vegetable oil
2 cups oats
1 teaspoon ground cinnamon
¼ cup butter
½ cup honey
1 cup brown sugar

Directions

1

Preheat oven to 350 degrees F.

2

Arrange apple slices in 9-inch circular glass pie plate.

3

Stir oats, brown sugar, and ground cinnamon together in a bowl.

4

Microwave butter in short 5-second increments until melted, about 20 seconds. Stir honey, melted butter, and oil into oat mixture; crumble over apples.

5

Bake in preheated oven until golden brown, about 35-40 minutes. Cool on a wire cooling rack, about 40-45 minutes.

Nutrition

Per Serving: 605 calories; protein 6g; carbohydrates 117.4g; fat 15.5g; cholesterol 30.5mg; sodium 97.4mg.

Yogurt Cheesecake

Prep:

20 mins

Cook:

15 mins

Additional:

3 hrs 5 mins

Total:

3 hrs 40 mins

Servings:

10

Yield:

1 10-inch cheesecake

Ingredients

For Crust:

½ cup butter

¼ cup packed dark brown sugar

¼ teaspoon sea salt

9 whole graham crackers

For Filling:

2 ½ teaspoons unflavored gelatin

3 (8 ounce) packages cream cheese, at room temperature

2 cups whole-milk Greek yogurt, at room temperature

1 tablespoon cold water

½ pinch white sugar

1 teaspoon lemon zest

1 pinch sea salt

1 teaspoon vanilla extract

1 tablespoon lemon juice

For Topping:

4 cups fresh blueberries

3 tablespoons packed dark brown sugar

1 teaspoon lemon zest

2 tablespoons lemon juice

Directions

1

Heat butter in a small saucepan over medium-low heat until it smells nutty and brown bits form on the bottom, about 16 minutes. Don't crank up the heat to try to get there faster; you'll just end up with burned butter.

2

Meanwhile, pulse together graham crackers, brown sugar, and salt in a food processor until fine crumbs form. Carefully pour butter into crumb mixture while food processor is running. Press combined mixture into bottom and sides of a 10-inch tart pan with a removable bottom. Chill for 1 hour or freeze for 20 minutes until set.

3

Stir together gelatin and cold water in a small bowl. Let stand for 5 minutes, then microwave until gelatin dissolves, about 10 seconds.

4

Beat cream cheese in a bowl with an electric mixer for 40 seconds. Add yogurt, white sugar, lemon juice, lemon zest, salt, and vanilla. Beat until smooth, then beat in gelatin. Pour mixture into the chilled crust. Chill until set, about 2 hours.

5

Stir together blueberries, brown sugar, poppy seeds, lemon juice, and lemon zest. Scatter topping over cheesecake.

Nutrition

Per Serving: 478 calories; protein 9.3g; carbohydrates 27g; fat 38.2g; cholesterol 107.3mg; sodium 409.3mg.

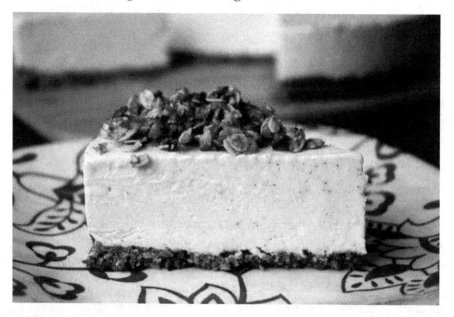

Peach Sorbet

Prep:

10 mins

Cook:

5 mins

Additional:

5 hrs 20 mins

Total:

5 hrs 35 mins

Servings:

8

Yield:

8 servings

Ingredients

2 tablespoons lemon juice

½ cup white sugar

½ cup water

1 pound ripe peaches - peeled, pitted, and chopped

Directions

1

Add peaches to a blender; blend until smooth. Measure out 1 1/2 cups peach puree into a bowl. Immediately stir in lemon juice and refrigerate.

2

Combine water and sugar in a small saucepan and bring to a boil. Stir until sugar is dissolved, about 1 minute. Remove from stove and cool to room temperature. Refrigerate simple syrup until chilled, about 1 hour.

3

Pour chilled peach puree and simple syrup into an ice cream maker and freeze according to manufacturer's instructions, about 20 minutes. Transfer to an airtight container and freeze until firm, about 4 hours.

Nutrition

Per Serving: 60 calories; carbohydrates 15.4g; sodium 2.2mg.

Strawberry Soufflè

Prep:

40 mins

Cook:

1 hr 15 mins

Total:

1 hr 55 mins

Servings:

10

Yield:

10 servings

Ingredients

4 large egg whites egg whites, at room temperature
Pinch salt
1 cup sugar
4 cups strawberries
1 tablespoon cornstarch
1 tablespoon white vinegar
¼ teaspoon cream of tartar
1 teaspoon vanilla
2 tablespoons orange liqueur
2 cups whipping cream

Directions

1

Beat egg whites, cream of tartar and salt in a large bowl with an electric mixer until soft peaks form. Beat in sugar, 1 tbsp at a time, until stiff, glossy peaks form. Beat in cornstarch, vinegar and vanilla just until blended.

2

On a baking sheet lined with parchment paper or foil, spread meringue into a 10-inch (25 cm) circle with a raised edge and a slight indentation in the centre.

3

Bake in a preheated 250 degrees F oven until firm to the touch, about 1-1/4 hours. Meringue should be cream-coloured. If it appears to be browning, reduce oven temperature to 225 degrees F.

4

Remove from oven and let cool.

5

When ready to serve, peel parchment paper off back of meringue. Place meringue on a serving plate. Cut strawberries into halves or slices, if large. Whip cream until stiff peaks form. Gently stir in liqueur, if using. Spread whipped cream over meringue leaving edge of meringue visible. Top with strawberries. Cut into wedges to serve.

Nutrition

Per Serving: 281 calories; protein 2.8g; carbohydrates 27.9g; fat 17.8g; cholesterol 65.2mg; sodium 41.2mg.

Pomegranate Granita

Prep:

10 mins

Total:

10 mins

Servings:

1

Yield:

1 cocktail

Ingredients

1 cup ice

2 teaspoons white sugar

1 (1.5 fluid ounce) jigger Cointreau or other orange liqueur

2 fluid ounces pomegranate syrup

1 orange slice

½ (1.5 fluid ounce) jigger white rum

Directions

1

Place the ice, Cointreau, rum, and pomegranate syrup into a blender, blend until smooth. Moisten the rim of a tumbler with the cut edge of the orange slice, and dip the glass into the sugar to line the rim. Pour the granita into the glass, and garnish with the orange slice to serve.

Nutrition

Per Serving: 387 calories; protein 0g; carbohydrates 66.4g; fat 0.1g; cholesterol 0mg; sodium 10.4mg.

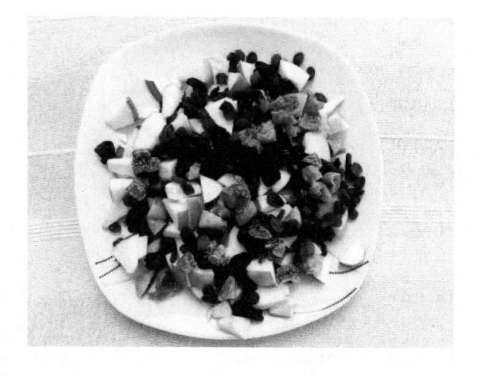